BECOMING A MIDWIFE

What is the reality of being a midwife in the twenty-first century? What is it like to help and support women throughout pregnancy and childbirth and into motherhood? What roles can midwives play in society?

This new edition of the popular text, *Becoming a Midwife*, explores what it is to be a midwife, looking at the factors that make midwifery such a special profession, as well as some of the challenges. The fully updated chapters cover a variety of settings and several different stages in a woman's pregnancy, including stories from midwives working in hospitals and in the community, as managers, supervisors and educators, and as men, women, mothers and birth activists. All chapters are narrated by contributors who introduce their own theme, recount a vignette that throws light on their understandings of midwifery and reasons for becoming (or not becoming) a midwife and any subsequent career moves. Backed up by commentaries and drawing together these insights, the editors show what it means to be a midwife today.

Suitable for those contemplating a career in midwifery and providing an opportunity for reflection for more experienced midwives, this thought-provoking book is an invaluable contribution to midwifery.

Rosemary Mander is Emeritus Professor of Midwifery at the University of Edinburgh, UK.

Valerie Fleming is Professor of Midwifery at the Zurich University of Applied Sciences, Switzerland.

BECOMING A MIDWIFE

Second edition

Edited by Rosemary Mander and Valerie Fleming

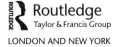

Routledge
Taylor & Francis Group

LONDON AND NEW YORK

First published 2009
by Routledge

This edition published 2014
by Routledge
2 Park Square, Milton Park, Abingdon, Oxon, OX14 4RN

and by Routledge
711 Third Avenue, New York, NY 10017

Routledge is an imprint of the Taylor & Francis Group, an informa business

British Library Cataloguing in Publication Data
A catalogue record for this book is available from the British Library

Library of Congress Cataloging in Publication Data
Becoming a midwife / edited by Rosemary Mander and Valerie Fleming – Second edition.
     p. cm.
  Includes bibliographical references.
  I. Mander, Rosemary, editor of compilation. II. Fleming, Valerie, editor of compilation. [DNLM: 1. Midwifery. 2. Career Choice. 3. Vocational Guidance. WQ 160]
  RG950
  618.2–dc23   2013045622

ISBN: 978-0-415-66009-9 (hbk)
ISBN: 978-0-415-66010-5 (pbk)
ISBN: 978-0-203-07436-7 (ebk)

Typeset in Bembo
by Keystroke, Station Road, Codsall, Wolverhampton

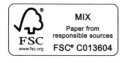

Printed and bound by CPI Group (UK) Ltd, Croydon, CR0 4YY

CONTENTS

CONTRIBUTORS

Penny Curtis I practised as a hospital-based midwife before moving to work in Central America, a move that radically changed my approach to birth. After returning to the UK, my doctoral research was fuelled by an interest in the ways that midwives work with, and relate to, women around birth within the bureaucratic setting of the hospital. Since then, my interests have broadly focused on social aspects of childbearing, parenting and family life and I have undertaken research in the areas of children's health and wellbeing. I currently hold a Chair in Child and Family Health and Wellbeing in the School of Nursing and Midwifery at the University of Sheffield.

Kirsty Darroch I recently qualified with distinction as a midwife in Glasgow and embarked upon my new career this year. With a background of more than 19 years in design and print, midwifery sees the fulfilment of a long-standing personal dream and a significant career change that I have embraced wholeheartedly. I now look forward to developing myself further as a midwife while continuing to pursue my other interests of writing children's stories, raising my two children and running.

Jean Duerden I spent the majority of my National Health Service (NHS) career in midwifery, throughout which I have had a passionate respect for the supervision of midwives. This ultimately led to my appointment as a Local Supervising Authority Midwifery Officer for Yorkshire and Northern Lincolnshire. Prior to taking on this role, I was involved in auditing the supervision of midwives both in the North and nationally. I have enjoyed writing about supervision, with publications in several professional journals and chapters on supervision in eight books, including the latest edition of Myles *Midwifery*. After retirement from the NHS and the LSA role I was lucky enough to continue meeting with the supervisors of midwives in the UK for whom I had a high regard by forming an event organising company to organise the biennial LSA Supervision Conferences in Nottingham.

Nadine Edwards I am a long-standing member of the Association for Improvements in the Maternity Services (AIMS) and am currently one of its Vice Chairs. I have run pregnancy groups since 1985 and set up birth educators' courses in the 1990s. I completed a PhD on women's experiences of planning home births in 2002 and have carried out research on women's experiences of being on Maternity Services Liaison Committees (MSLC), and the experiences of women who withdraw from maternity services during their pregnancies, and give birth without midwives. I commissioned articles for and contributed to *Essentially MIDIRS*, and was recently the co-editor of the *MIDIRS Midwifery Digest*. I continue to research, write and lecture on various aspects of birth and midwifery.

Allison Ewing I qualified as a midwife in 1988 and was lucky enough to work in one of the Riverside Midwifery Teams in London for 5 years, working as a truly autonomous midwifery practitioner within the NHS. Having then been even luckier to experience true continuity of carer from a trusted friend and colleague when I had my first baby, I was inspired to want to work as a caseloading midwife. Unfortunately, when I returned to Scotland in 1996, there was no such model of care available (and there still isn't) so in order to provide that continuity I became an independent midwife. I had hoped to be able to continue in clinical practice in this way till retirement but (at the time of writing) EU legislation has been temporarily shelved with a view to enactment in February 2014, which will stop me providing care for women labouring at home. I have been an active member of the Independent Midwives of the United Kingdom and served on the board for several years. I have had several articles published in *Midwifery Matters*, the journal of the Association of Radical Midwives. In the past, I have served as a steward for the Royal College of Midwives, but with great sadness, I will be resigning from that organisation in the near future in order to access insurance from the Royal College of Nursing.

Valerie Fleming Becoming a midwife was my gateway to the world although I was not aware of that at the time. The cruise ship on which I wanted to be a nurse told me I had to be a midwife as well as obtain a whole host of other qualifications. I decided to see the world while getting these qualifications and that led to midwifery practice first in India and then New Zealand. I must have been a slow learner because I did not progress past my 16 years in New Zealand, instead finding a rewarding career in hospital then community midwifery and finally in the academic world. The opportunity to be active in World Health Organisation projects brought me back to Scotland where I was based for a further 16 years before moving first to Denmark and then Switzerland. I now work as a Professor of Midwifery at Zurich University of Applied Sciences.

Yvonne Fontein I was born in the Netherlands where I worked in maternity care as an obstetric nurse before moving to Scotland to become a midwife. After qualifying I moved back to the Netherlands and worked there as a community-based independent midwife for 8 years, where I supported many women in labouring and giving birth in their own homes. I continued studying at Glasgow Caledonian University (GCU) and after graduating with an MSc in midwifery I worked at GCU as a lecturer. Nowadays I am once more in the Netherlands where I combine research with teaching and with work in the labour ward. Additionally, I occasionally practise as an independent midwife.

Eleanor Forrest I was born and brought up in Scotland and educated as a nurse and midwife in Glasgow. Over the past 30 years I have lived and worked in a variety of countries and midwifery environments. My Master of Philosophy was about women's experiences and perceptions of service provision for women experiencing postnatal depression. Much of my clinical experience as a midwife has focused on providing holistic care to women with mental health problems and their families during the perinatal period. I was the first midwife to provide a specialist service that provides for childbearing women with perinatal mental health problems in Glasgow. Through working with women in this capacity I have recognised that adaptation to motherhood often involves a process of loss and grieving, as women change the focus of their lives. Currently, I work as a lecturer in midwifery at Glasgow Caledonian University. I am involved in delivering modules I have written for multi-professional perinatal mental health practitioners. I also lecture on the undergraduate midwifery programme and deliver international postgraduate Master's modules using a virtual learning environment. I have recently co-written the book *Bereavement Care for Childbearing Women and their Families*. I occasionally practise as an independent midwife.

Elaine Haycock-Stuart I undertook my nursing and midwifery education in Yorkshire in the 1980s prior to moving to Scotland where I worked as a midwife before undertaking a health visitor programme there. After several years in health visiting practice I undertook research projects and my PhD at the University of Edinburgh. I commenced lecturing at the University of Stirling prior to taking up a lectureship in 2002 in Nursing Studies at the University of Edinburgh where I now work as a Senior Lecturer and Director of Learning and Teaching. I am married and have one wonderful daughter.

Ans Luyben I was born, brought up and trained as a midwife and a teacher in the Netherlands. I worked as a midwife, teacher/lecturer and researcher in institutions in the Netherlands as well as in Switzerland. My PhD addressed care during pregnancy from women's points of view in Switzerland, the Netherlands and Scotland. Currently, I work as a midwife in the hospital Spital STS AG in Thun, where I am involved in practice development. I have carried out several research projects and published on a variety of midwifery subjects in German, French,

Dutch and English. My research interests involve person-centred practice, antenatal care, models of care provision, education and cross-national comparative studies.

Nessa McHugh I qualified as a midwife in 1990 and since then have worked in the NHS, education and carried a small caseload as an independent midwife. I am currently a midwifery lecturer in Scotland where I have also practised as an independent midwife. I am also a supervisor of midwives and I am interested in all things midwifery, especially feminism, relational midwifery practice and supporting midwives to support women.

Carrie McIntosh I live in Bonnyrigg, near Edinburgh, with my husband, three children, two dogs and six chickens. After working in hospitality and medically-related jobs and facing redundancy, my interest in midwifery was aroused by an advert for a midwifery programme. Lacking confidence, I put this idea to one side, but the desire re-emerged after having my first baby. Due to the fantastic midwives who had cared for me, my childbearing experience had empowered me and I felt, "if I can do that, I can do anything!" But it was another 6 years before I was to begin my midwifery. I trained with an amazing team of inspirational community midwives who taught me what it was to truly care for women and to trust in birth, women and their bodies. As if I didn't have enough to contend with immediately after qualifying, I was surprised to find that I was expecting my third baby. Everything fell into place and I found that I was able to juggle all of the demands relatively easily. Seven years on, I have continued to practise as an independent midwife, whilst also working on the bank for two local trusts.

Rosemary Mander Practising as a midwife encouraged me to move into midwifery teaching and then higher education in the University of Edinburgh. My doctoral studies arose from my observation of poor retention of newly qualified midwives; an interest in labour force issues continues. My interests have moved towards the politics of maternity care, including historical and international aspects. These feature a strong woman–centred orientation, including both the childbearing woman and the woman as a midwife. Until recently I continued regular practice as a midwife under an honorary appointment with Lothian Health and have practised independently.

Miranda Page I was born in Nigeria but was brought up in numerous locations throughout the UK. After finishing a BA (Hons) in history and drama I sought fame and fortune in London working for 6 years in the retail trade – Harrods. Being not completely satisfied with this career choice I packed my car and moved to a remote island off the west coast of Scotland. Iona provided the inspiration for my final career change (to date), and thinking that midwifery would offer me the opportunity to do something important and travel the world I moved to Edinburgh and never left. Midwifery has been my longest career though I have explored different aspects of it. In 2000 I gained an MSc in Nursing Studies from the

University of Edinburgh and 10 years later, after working in a busy labour ward, a PhD from Queen Margaret University Edinburgh. Now my interest lies in postnatal care from a practice and research perspective. I am currently a Clinical Research Fellow in the NMAHP Research Unit in the University of Stirling where they are attempting to re-design postnatal care.

Denis Walsh I was born and brought up in Queensland, Australia, but trained as a midwife in Leicester, UK and have worked in a variety of midwifery environments over the past 25 years. My PhD was on the Birth Centre model and I am now Associate Professor in Midwifery at the University of Nottingham. I lecture on evidence and skills for normal birth internationally and am widely published on midwifery issues and normal birth. I authored the best seller *Evidence-Based Care for Normal Labour and Birth*.

ABBREVIATIONS

ARM   artificial rupture of membranes (see Glossary)
ARM   Association of Radical Midwives
CEMACH   Confidential Enquiry into Maternal and Child Health
CEMD   Confidential Enquiry into Maternal Deaths
CIS   Commonwealth of Independent States
CTG   cardiotocograph (see Glossary)
DFID   Department for International Development
EEC   European Economic Community
EPDS   Edinburgh Postnatal Depression Scale
EU   European Union
EWTD   European Working Time Directive
FGM   female genital mutilation
FIGO   Federation International of Gynecology and Obstetrics
GP   general practitioner
HDU   high-dependency unit (see Glossary)
HE   higher education
ICM   International Confederation of Midwives
IMA   Independent Midwives Association
LSA   Local Supervising Authority
LSAMO   Local Supervising Authority Midwifery Officer
ME   myalgic encephalomyelitis (see Glossary)
MSLC   Maternity Service Liaison Committee
NHS   National Health Service
NICE   National Institute for Health and Clinical Excellence
NIVEL   Netherlands Institute for Health Services Research
NMC   Nursing and Midwifery Council
NQM   newly qualified midwife

OP	occipito-posterior position (see Glossary)
PBL	problem-based learning
PII	professional indemnity insurance
PND	postnatal depression
PPH	post-partum haemorrhage (see Glossary)
RCM	Royal College of Midwives
SIGN	Scottish Intercollegiate Guidelines Network
UCAS	Universities and Colleges Admissions Service in the UK
UK	United Kingdom
UN	United Nations
USA	United States of America
VBAC	vaginal birth after Caesarean
VSO	Voluntary Service Overseas
WHO	World Health Organization
WHOCC	World Health Organization Collaborating Centre

INTRODUCTION

Choosing midwifery and being a midwife

Rosemary Mander and Valerie Fleming

Through the medium of this book, we are endeavouring to explore the nature and the meaning of midwifery for and to the midwife. It is our intention that this exploration will be of value to two rather different groups of people who are contemplating midwifery. On the one hand, you may be musing on midwifery because you are considering entering it with a view to making your career as a midwife; this may be either as a first career or as a career change later in your life. On the other hand, you may be an experienced and highly expert midwife who is taking an opportunity to reflect on your future career with a view to deciding whether to stay in midwifery and, if so, in which area. This book is written with the intention of providing food for thought that will assist both groups in making these crucially important life choices.

When writing about midwifery, authors tend to accentuate the positives. This is entirely understandable because, as an occupation, when midwifery is good it is very good. As the experienced midwife will admit and as some midwifery students may have learned during their programme, though, this rose-tinted view may not convey the complete picture. In order to achieve the aims of this book, it is fundamentally important that we provide an honest representation of what midwifery is about. Were this not the case, the experienced midwife would rightly dismiss this book as, at best, a joke and, at worst, a deceit. A midwifery student lulled into such naïve complacency would be rightfully angry at such trickery. Thus, with these readers and their differing requirements in mind, we are striving to present an honest portrayal of midwifery as an occupation in the early twenty-first century. The image which we offer may not necessarily accord with the views and experiences of some midwives, as they are a quite heterogeneous group. It will, however, comprise a realistic, but not necessarily flattering, portrait which will serve to stimulate questioning and facilitate serious deliberation.

The second edition

The need for a further edition of this book reflects a number of changes, both in midwifery and in the social and health environments of which midwifery practice is a part. So the question needs to be answered about what has changed since the first edition was published in 2009. As well as all of us growing at least 5 years older, there have been a number of developments with implications for the midwife and for midwifery.

In the UK, at least, there has been a veritable welter of media outpourings, regaling us with romanticised and nostalgic views of midwifery in times past (Worth 2007; Light 2011; Anderson 2012; Byrom 2011; Fairley 2012). The rose-tinted spectacles alluded to above appear to have gone into overdrive with such a media frenzy. This furore may be attributable to a belated knock-on effect from the sixtieth anniversary celebrations on the birth of the UK NHS, the diamond jubilee or to television producers' love affair with costume dramas. The effect of this 'sanitised' representation of reality (Brintworth in Dabrowski 2012), though, is not totally benign, as such idealised depictions may give rise to disillusionment among childbearing women hoping for deeply personalised continuity of care.

A further aspect of this media overdrive has been found in television programmes which feature a 'fly on the wall' approach. The first, *One Born Every Minute*, was set in an English labour suite (Channel 4 2011). Although widely acclaimed for its sympathetic honesty, Henrietta Otley argues that it may cause 'performance anxiety' to become as counterproductive in childbearing as it is in other fields of human activity (2012). Otley considers this difficulty for women, but neglects to mention that the same difficulty may also apply to the midwife's practice.

In historical terms, through most of the twentieth century, UK midwifery took a certain pride in the light touch of its regulatory system, although this may have turned to despair in recent times. Statutory regulation has been discredited by first the United Kingdom Central Council for Nursing, Midwifery and Health Visiting (UKCC) and, more recently, by its replacement organisation the Nursing and Midwifery Council (NMC).

Statutory regulation by the NMC has been shown to have totally disgraced some honourable occupational groups, such as independent midwives. This was demonstrated through the NMC having been investigated by the Council for Healthcare Regulatory Excellence (CHRE), which is a super-regulator brought in to resolve public distrust following a series of scandals involving medical practitioners. The final report of the CHRE (2012) recommended 15 changes, which are intended to deal with shortcomings affecting leadership, culture, finance and operational management. Most tellingly, the CHRE identified a passive, hierarchical culture of 'resigned resilience', through which NMC staff became frustrated at their own inability to remedy this quango's dysfunctional organisation (Bird 2012). Disappointingly, the CHRE report resorted to recommending the time-honoured yet singularly ineffectual panacea of 'leadership'; this, the CHRE naïvely anticipated, will introduce a culture change in the NMC to restore the confidence of all who are involved.

Far from unrelated to the debacle which is UK midwifery's statutory regulation is the threat of annihilation to one particular group of midwives, who are widely perceived as torch-bearers for woman-oriented midwifery care. These are the midwives who I am calling 'independent midwives' (see Chapter 10) who practise outside the regulated, obstetric-dominated, state systems of maternity care, offering women a continuity and freedom of choice which is otherwise unavailable. This process of obliteration is well established in the United States, having been initiated to resolve the 'midwife problem' in the opening years of the twentieth century (Davis-Floyd & Bonaro 2012). More recently the death-knell for UK independent midwifery was sounded when the membership of the Royal College of Midwives declined to support its independent co-professionals in the provision of professional indemnity insurance (Warren 1994). What has become known as a 'witch hunt' has involved the NMC in cases such as that of Becky Reed (2012). A similar situation is manifesting itself in the Republic of Ireland through the new legislation (ISB 2011) which grants the midwife the recognition as distinct from nurses, which has so long been sought. The obverse side of this particular coin is found in the requirement that the self-employed community, or independent, midwife (SECM) is now under threat of a devastating financial penalty and/or imprisonment if attending at home a woman whose characteristics do not conform with strict criteria; for example, an SECM may not attend a woman at home who has previously undergone a caesarean. Jo Murphy-Lawless summarises the effects of this legislation as 'a disaster for Irish midwifery and for women' (2012:69).

Amid this gloomy global scenario, a particular candle which has continued to illuminate a woeful world also appears to be wavering. In the Netherlands, according to Marian van Huis (2012), the midwife's autonomy has effectively been curtailed. Tighter medical control now constrains her practice, in the form of a more stringent Indications List (VIL 1999).

In the UK the overwhelming majority of midwives who practise are employed within the National Health Service (NHS), which has been undergoing many changes, and of which more are threatened. A range of recent developments in the NHS have resulted in an increasing commercialisation of health care in general and of maternity in particular. This conversion of health care to a market orientation has been associated with women's reduced access to some services (Mander 2011).

The forthcoming changes to the NHS in England (TSO 2012) have aggravated fears of escalating commercialisation (Reynolds & McKee 2012). These fears have centred on the requirement for services to be offered by 'Any qualified provider', which is the revised version of the original 'Any willing provider' (Dearden-Phillips 2011). The likelihood is that gigantic commercial corporations will seize this opportunity to increase their profits, by diverting public sector funds. The only beneficiaries of this process will be the corporate directors and shareholders. The small organisations, such as charities, and the communities which they serve, will be left having to fend for themselves.

Choosing midwifery

Against this backdrop of a changing context, both in terms of public perceptions and organisations, decisions are being made about entering, continuing and, possibly, leaving midwifery. These decisions are momentous. They affect the health care system, the midwifery profession, childbearing women and their families and, not least, the would-be, newly qualified or experienced midwife who is making the decision. The choice of entering or staying in midwifery is likely to be determined by personal experience.

For the qualified midwife who has been in practice, the decision will be between three possibilities. First is staying put as a, possibly clinical, practitioner. Second is moving into another, non-clinical, area of midwifery such as research, management or teaching. The third possibility is leaving midwifery, perhaps to move into a related area, or else to break away into a totally different sphere.

The decision to become a midwifery student and then a midwife is also likely to be based on experience. For a small number this experience will have been gained during a nursing programme. For more would-be midwifery students, it is personal experience obtained through childbearing which determines the decision. For others the experience may be gained less directly through another's child-bearing or through non-professional personal contact with a midwife or midwives.

Thus, it is clear that it is necessary for a decision to be made in which com-parisons are drawn on the basis of a wide range of information. It is our intention that this book will contribute to the information-gathering which contributes to the midwifery practice decision.

Midwifery as a practice discipline

In the first edition, while exploring midwifery from a number of different viewpoints, we emphasised the importance of midwifery being a practice discipline. This focus has, if anything, become even more significant since the first edition was published. It is possible that this emphasis on practice has become apparent through the midwife's usual attention to those for whom care is provided, that is, the childbearing woman and her family. This focus, it may be suggested, has been at the expense of the midwife's consideration of their own behaviour and activities. Thus, less is written about the way in which the midwife views midwifery in general and her own role in particular. Such midwifery self-neglect, though, is to be corrected through this book which, quite explicitly and unashamedly, concentrates on the midwife and the midwife's views of midwifery practice and the environment in which midwifery practice happens. This is because the factor which is consistent throughout midwifery is the fundamental nature of midwifery as a form of practice. The sole *raison d'être* for the many aspects of midwifery relate, if they are to maintain credibility, to practice. Although aspects such as management decision making or theory building may consume the time of midwife managers and academics, if they have no bearing on practice they become futile. Further, there may be any number of ways of approaching, analysing or explaining midwifery, but they all come down to the primacy of the actual activities or behaviour of the midwife in relation to the childbearing woman, which materialise in the process of attending that woman. In spite of all the technological and other developments in maternity care, it is the practice of the midwife that continues to provide the crucial focus for all those involved in midwifery. The quintessential nature of practice is clearly apparent in the, possibly somewhat limited, definition of a midwife drawn up by the International Confederation of Midwives (ICM) (WHO/ICM/FIGO 2005):

> A midwife is a person who, having been regularly admitted to a midwifery educational programme, duly recognised in the country in which it is located, has successfully completed the prescribed course of studies in midwifery and has acquired the requisite qualifications to be registered and/or legally licensed to practise midwifery.

> The midwife is recognised as a responsible and accountable professional who works in partnership with women to give the necessary support, care and advice during pregnancy, labour and the postpartum period, to conduct births on the midwife's own responsibility and to provide care for the newborn and the infant. This care includes preventative measures, the promotion of normal birth, the detection of complications in mother and child, the accessing of medical care or other appropriate assistance and the carrying out of emergency measures.

> The midwife has an important task in health counselling and education, not only for the woman, but also within the family and the community. This work should involve antenatal education and preparation for parenthood and may extend to women's health, sexual or reproductive health and child care.

> A midwife may practise in any setting including the home, community, hospitals, clinics or health units.

Although the focus on and centrality of midwifery practice are unalterable, that practice and the related activities are most certainly not. The practice environment will, to a large extent and in many different ways, facilitate the practice of the midwife. On those occasions when the environment may not actually be facilitatory, it continues to be otherwise influential. In this way the midwife interacts with and responds to the phenomena by which she is surrounded. Examples of these phenomena would include the consumer's and the medical inputs into maternity services. Similarly, the midwife may select the value which she attaches to the plethora of technological devices and decide whether and when she employs them in her practice. The same degree of selectivity would apply to the midwife's use of the research evidence base with which she needs to be familiar and which may serve to facilitate more effective midwifery practice. The result of this constant interaction between midwife and the childbearing environment is the development of a midwifery system. This interaction is in a constant state of flux, with factors changing through increasing or declining significance. Thus, we should regard the midwifery system as dynamic, in that it is constantly adjusting and readjusting with regard to this multiplicity of developments. Some of these adjustments may be purely reactive, in response to changes in, for example, the aspirations of those for whom the midwife provides care. A large proportion of innovative practices, though, will be introduced proactively through the advance of new ideas, research and novel ways of thinking.

For many reasons, including the midwife's interaction with the environment mentioned already, attention to perceptions of the midwife's role has also been shown to be necessary. Uncertainty about the midwifery role is widespread, as those of us who have often bridled at being addressed as 'nurse' can attest. We would like to think that this necessity and any uncertainty may have been addressed by midwifery's recent media exposure (see above), but this may not be the case. While the media attention may have persuaded the public, as viewers and readers, of what the midwife is capable of, there remain others still needing to be convinced. Nurses, to whom some may consider the midwife to be related, have long encountered difficulty in understanding why and how midwifery is different (Mander 2008). This incomprehension was opened up for debate (Norman & Griffiths 2007) and more recent publications show that it continues to bother nurses (Griffiths & Norman 2011). Our medical colleagues are known to encounter similar difficulties, which have been articulated by Jim Dornan (2008). It may be suggested that both occupational groups suffer an arrogant form of myopia, which prevents their male-dominated academic leadership from recognising midwifery's woman- and community-oriented underpinnings. Whether and to what extent such uncertainty about the midwife's role features among midwives is in urgent need of attention; this is partly because of the existence of that hybrid, the medical midwife or 'medwife', which has been advanced in another country with limited recent midwifery authority (Davis-Floyd *et al.* 2010).

The decision to choose to either enter or remain in midwifery clearly has significant implications, but not only for the midwife. Those who are nearest and dearest to the potential or actual midwife also deserve careful attention. These significant others are likely to include partners in long-term relationships as well as any existing or yet-to-be-born children. The commitment which is particularly demanded of certain groups of midwives may not be easily compatible with conventional views of both family and social life. Examples are likely to include the challenges faced by the independent midwife, the caseloading midwife (see below) and, possibly, the global midwife. Thus, certain groups may find themselves having to think very carefully about their priorities before embarking on the career path of their choice.

Decisions: What it has not been possible to include

This book endeavours to explore the authors' understanding of the meaning of midwifery. Because midwifery, as explained already, and the midwife's role are dynamic, there are many aspects. It has not been possible to address all of these aspects, so some selectivity has been necessary. We have needed to omit some aspects, which may be considered to be relevant. In this section we mention a few of these omissions and our reasons for reaching these challenging decisions.

First, it is essential to recall that midwifery, as an occupational group, has evolved and is continuing to do so. This is partly in response to the aspirations of child-bearing women and also to the health care environment within which most midwives practise. One of the spin-offs resulting from this evolution is the change in or fragmentation of the role of the midwife into a plethora of specialist roles. This multiplicity of roles may be regarded as demonstrating the midwife's responsiveness to the twenty-first century milieu. An alternative interpretation, though, is that the midwife may be being forced to lose sight of the individual childbearing woman in the interests of focusing on the problems which the woman may face and which are of less interest to other health care providers.

This process of occupational change represents a supreme example of a phenomenon familiar in many professions and other jobs, including nursing (Read 2004), known as role extension. Susan Read's argument is surprisingly relevant to midwifery, as she outlines the potential for roles to be extended in a mechanistic manner for organisational purposes; her apposite example is the role changes imposed on a number of health care occupations following the enactment of the European Working Time Directive (EWTD) (European Union 1993). Such short-sighted changes carry risks affecting both staff and recipients of care, in the form of staff burnout. The preferred route to the development of roles is the more organic pathway which being more humane and, hence, healthier, is known as role expansion.

The specialist midwifery roles include those focusing on drug/alcohol misuse, infant feeding, bereavement, ultrasound diagnosis, mental health, teenage preg-nancy, smoking cessation, domestic violence, screening in pregnancy, clinical governance/risk, child protection, diabetes mellitus, obesity, multiple pregnancy, HIV/AIDS, blood dyscrasias, female genital mutilation, epilepsy, infertility, homelessness, preconception and disadvantaged women (Hawkins 2006). While some of these roles have been shown to be associated with demonstrably better outcomes, the impression of benefits for the woman and/or baby is far from unambiguous (Caird *et al.* 2010). On the other hand, Abigail Masterson admits that the seamless and unfragmented form of midwifery care associated with continuity of carer is much appreciated by women (2010). The fact that, as she recognises, this form of care is more difficult to actually achieve may mean that such aspirations are doomed.

The second, not unrelated, aspect which is unable to be a focus of attention is midwife-led care in its various forms. Categorisation of these forms is not easy due to the variations in organisation and terminology, but they share a common theoretical underpinning in striving for continuity of care/r to facilitate uncomplicated birth experiences for the healthy childbearing woman. The midwife is the lead health care provider, practising in a partnership with the woman who is regarded as enjoying a 'low-risk' childbearing experience. While a community orientation is often assumed, midwife-led care may happen in maternity units as well as alongside and in freestanding birthing centres (Walsh & Devane 2012). The midwives offering these forms of care may practise as a, hopefully, small number forming a 'group' or 'team'. A more refined version of care is known as 'caseload' practice, when care is provided by one midwife, with support from another (Hatem *et al.* 2008).

Although it has attracted attention in other areas, some years have passed since the maternity team has been of interest (Kitzinger *et al.* 1990). In view of the uncertain existence of the interprofessional clinical team, it is probably better if there is no further mention.

In maternity as well as many other aspects of enterprise, leadership has long been presented as some kind of organisational panacea. It may be argued that the nature, reality and effectiveness of leadership are questionable. More pragmatically, leadership is appropriately regarded as situational, therefore the potential for leadership resides within the individual midwife (Lynch *et al.* 2011).

A clinician whose presence features prominently in many maternity services, albeit with different titles, is the maternity care assistant (MCA). Also known as the maternity support worker (MSW), maternity health care assistant, health care assistant, auxiliary nurse or maternity aid (Hussain & Marshall 2011; Browne 2005; Jones & Jenkins 2004:60; Davies 2009; van Teijlingen 1994), this health care worker, we are reassured, works only under a midwife's supervision and undertakes only delegated tasks (Hussain & Marshall 2011; Rennie *et al.* 2009). The increasing significance of this worker's input is likely to be a 'knock-on' effect of the European Working Time Directive (DoH 1998). Despite the supervision and delegation restrictions, Catriona Hussain and Jayne Marshall report confusion about the precise nature of the MCA's roles. These authors articulate concerns about further erosion of the midwife's role and whether she is able to remain accountable for fulfilling her statutory responsibilities. Hussain and Marshall's warning to midwives is opportune, stating that they need to 'be advocates for the midwifery profession by questioning current practice and challenging new developments in the workplace' (2011:340).

The final group of midwives to whom this book is not able to give the attention which they deserve, are those unable to find midwifery employment and are, thus, unemployed. In the UK this phenomenon may be affected by changes in education and demographics, resulting in the newly qualified midwife being less able to move to a different area to find midwifery employment. An on-line search of midwifery vacancies, though, found them to take the form of international permanent posts only, with some temporary posts advertised for the south-east of England. The existence of a shortage of posts is reported to have been recognised by the RCM

(Editorial 2012). On an international basis it is more difficult to separate midwifery unemployment from figures for nurses, in the WHO data demonstrating a global shortage (2010) and other authoritative data (Bloor & Maynard 2003). Like much of the UK, though, the economic downturn has been blamed for the worst affected countries, such as Spain, Greece and Italy, seeking to reduce or downsize their nursing workforce. Because of the similarities in employment, it is probably safe to surmise that a similar process is affecting midwifery (Alameddine *et al.* 2012). Even more alarming, though, are the data which show that those countries with the lowest numbers in proportion to the population size, such as Spain, Portugal and 'Korea', are the countries most actively downsizing to reduce those numbers (Buchan & Black 2011).

The arrangement of the chapters in this book

With the assistance of real-life vignettes, each chapter will focus on a different aspect of midwifery. In this way the factors that generate dynamism within midwifery will emerge. Through each contributor's reflection on the experience-based vignette that she or he has chosen to recount, it will become clear what it was that brought the person to enter or not enter midwifery in the first place. Of course, this may or may not be the same as what encourages the midwife to remain in midwifery. Through these reflections, what will manifest itself is the meaning of midwifery to the midwife who practises it.

The editors' commentaries, summaries and reflections will serve to draw out the linkages and themes that happen to unite the chapters by the very different individuals who are the contributors. In this way the book will achieve its first purpose, which is to highlight, for the potential student or newly qualified midwife, the career opportunities that are likely to present themselves. Also provided will be much food for thought, which may need to be considered before embarking on this new career. As well as providing a guide for the new midwife, this book will also offer an opportunity for the more experienced and expert midwife to undertake a 'reality check'. This will facilitate reflection on the position of the expert midwife and of midwifery in the wider health care system and in the world as a whole. Such reflection is likely to assist practitioners and others in making decisions about their future career development.

The first part of the book concentrates on those aspects of the midwifery role that are probably of most interest to someone contemplating a midwifery career. As well as studying midwifery, this part addresses characteristics of midwifery that relate to working with women in an institution, such as a National Health Service (NHS) setting. In order to emphasise the needs of the potential midwife, the first part will be organised chronologically.

The second part of the book looks at aspects of midwifery that are not so widely known. These aspects will be addressed in order to demonstrate aspects which should be considered by those entering midwifery. This material is also likely to be valuable to the more experienced midwife contemplating career development.

There will also be an attempt to address the issues raised by these roles. In order to broaden the reader's horizons, the international orientation will be more pronounced in the second part.

References

Alameddine, M., Baumann, A., Laporte, A. and Deber, R. (2012) 'A narrative review on the effect of economic downturns on the nursing labour market: implications for policy and planning'. *Human Resources for Health* 10(23). http://www.human-resources-health.com/content/10/1/23

Anderson, M. (2012) *Tales of a Midwife*. London: Headline.

Bird, H. (2012) 'No more chances'. *Midwives* 15(5): 38–40.

Bloor, K. & Maynard, A. (2003) 'Planning human resources in health care: Towards an economic approach. An international comparative review'. Canadian Health Services Research Foundation Ottawa. http://www.cfhi-fcass.ca/Migrated/PDF/Research Reports/CommissionedResearch/bloor_e.pdf. Accessed January 2013.

Browne, A. (2005) 'Education and training of the maternity care assistant: developments from a BTEC diploma in maternity care'. *RCM Midwives*, 8(2): 72–3.

Buchan, J. & Black, S. (2011) 'The impact of pay increases on nurses' labour market: a review of evidence from four OECD countries'. OECD Health Working Papers, No. 57 OECD Publishing. http://dx.doi.org/10.1787/5kg6jwn16tjd-en.

Byrom, S. (2011) *Catching Babies: A Midwife's Tale*. London: Headline.

Caird, J., Rees, R., Kavanagh, J., Sutcliffe, K., Oliver, K., Dickson, K., Woodman, J., Barnett-Page, E. and Thomas, J. (2010) *The Socioeconomic Value of Nursing and Midwifery: A Rapid Systematic Review of Reviews*. EPPI Centre, Social Science Research Unit, Institute of Education, University of London, London.

Channel 4 (2011) *One Born Every Minute*. http://lifebegins.channel4.com/. Accessed January 2013.

CHRE (2012) *Strategic Review of the Nursing and Midwifery Council Final Report*, 3 July 2012. Council for Healthcare Regulatory Excellence. https://www.chre.org.uk/_img/pics/library/120702_CHRE_Final_Report_for_NMC_strategic_review_(pdf)_1.pdf. Accessed November 2012.

Dabrowski, R. (2012) 'The impact of drama'. *Midwives* 15(3): 38–40.

Davies, S. (2009) 'Jury of your peers?' *AIMS Journal* 21(3): 10–11.

Davis-Floyd, R. and Pascali Bonaro (sic), D. (2012) Joint letter to participants. Presented at Human Rights in Childbirth Conference International Conference of Jurists, Midwives & Obstetricians 61–3, The Hague.

Davis-Floyd, R., Pascal-Bonaro, D., Davies, R. and Gomez Ponce de Leon, R. (2010) 'The International Motherbaby Childbirth Initiative: A human rights approach to optimal maternity care'. *Midwifery Today* 94 Summer.

Dearden-Phillips, C. (2011) 'How will the Any Willing Provider model affect public services?' *Guardian*, 7 March. http://www.guardian.co.uk/public-leaders-network/2011/mar/07/any-willing-provider-public-services. Accessed November 2012.

DoH (1998) European Working Time Directive London. http://webarchive.national archives.gov.uk/+/www.dh.gov.uk/en/Managingyourorganisation/Workforce/Work forceplanninganddevelopment/Europeanworkingtimedirective/index.htm. Accessed October 2011.

Dornan, J. (2008) 'Is childbirth in the UK really mother centred?' *International Journal of Nursing Studies*, 45(6): 809–11.

Editorial (2012) 'Newly qualified midwives struggle to find jobs'. *Practising Midwife*, 15(11): 6.

European Union (1993) European Working Time Directive. http://www.eu-working-directive.co.uk/. Accessed January 2013.

Fairley, L. (2012) *The Midwife's Here: The Enchanting True Story of One of Britain's Longest Serving Midwives.* London: Harper Element.

Griffiths, P. and Norman, I. (2011) 'What is a nursing research journal?' *International Journal of Nursing Studies* 48(11): 1311–4.

Hatem, M., Sandall, J., Devane, D., Soltani, H. and Gates, S. (2008) *Midwife-led Versus Other Models of Care for Childbearing Women.* Cochrane Database of Systematic Reviews 2008, Issue 4. Art. No.: CD004667. doi: 10.1002/14651858.CD004667.pub2.

Hawkins, J. (2006) *Annual Report of Supervision of Midwives and Midwifery Practice South Yorkshire 2005–2006.* http://www.nmc-uk.org/Documents/Midwifery-LSA-reports/LSA%20Annual%20Report%20South%20Yorkshire%202005%202006.pdf. Accessed January 2013.

Hussain, C.J. and Marshall, J.E. (2011) 'The effect of the developing role of the maternity support worker on the professional accountability of the midwife'. *Midwifery* 27(3): 336–41.

ISB (2011) *Nurses and Midwives Act Number 41*, Irish Statute Book. http://www.irishstatutebook.ie/2011/en/act/pub/0041/index.html. Accessed May 2012.

Jones, S.R. & Jenkins, R. (2004) *The Law and the Midwife.* Oxford: Blackwell.

Kitzinger, J., Green, J. and Coupland, V. (1990) 'Labour relations', in J. Garcia, R. Kilpatrick, and M. Richards, *The Politics of Maternity Care: Services for Childbearing Women in Twentieth-Century Britain.* Oxford: Clarendon, pp. 149–62.

Light, A. (2011) *Midwife on Call: Tales of Tiny Miracles.* London: Hodder & Stoughton.

Lynch, B.M., McCormack, B. and McCance, T. (2011) 'Development of a model of situational leadership in residential care for older people'. *Journal of Nursing Management* 19(8): 1058–69. doi:10.1111/j.1365-

Mander, R. (2008) 'Extricating midwifery from the elephant's bed'. *International Journal of Nursing Studies* 45(5): 649–53.

Mander, R. (2011) 'Commercialisation and entrepreneurialism in maternity services'. *Midwifery* 27(4): 393–8.

Masterson, A. (2010) *Final Report Core and Developing Role of the Midwife: Literature Review.* http://midwifery2020.org/documents/2020/Core_Role_Lit_review.pdf. Accessed May 2012.

Murphy-Lawless, J. (2012) 'Empty promises: the dangers of risk discourses'. Presented at Human Rights in Childbirth Conference International Conference of Jurists, Midwives & Obstetricians 68–73, The Hague.

Norman, I. and Griffiths, P. (2007) '". . . And midwifery": time for a parting of the ways or a closer union with nursing?' *International Journal of Nursing Studies* 44(4): 521–2 (doi:10.1016/j.ijnurstu.2007.03.003).

Otley, H. (2012) 'One born every minute: mothers' performance anxiety'. *Practising Midwife* 15(2): 25–6.

Read, S. (2004) 'New nursing roles: Deciding the future for Scotland. Exploring role development and role expansion – is there a difference and does it matter?' Scottish Government. http://www.scotland.gov.uk/Publications/2004/04/19201/35582. Accessed January 2013.

Reed, B. (2012) 'A midwife under investigation'. Presented at Human Rights in Childbirth Conference International Conference of Jurists, Midwives & Obstetricians 116–7, The Hague.

Rennie, A.M., Gibb, S., Hourston, A., Bedford, H. and McNicol, J. (2009) 'The development of maternity care assistants in Scotland'. *Practising Midwife* 12(8): 14, 16–9.

Reynolds, L. and McKee, M. (2012) '"Any qualified provider" in NHS reforms: but who will qualify?' *Lancet* 379(9821): 1083–4.

TSO (2012) *Health and Social Care Act*. London: The Stationery Office. http://www.legislation.gov.uk/ukpga/2012/7/contents. Accessed November 2012.

van Huis, M. (2012) 'Home birth through the ages'. Presented at Human Rights in Childbirth Conference International Conference of Jurists, Midwives & Obstetricians 152–5, The Hague.

van Teijlingen, E.R. (1994) 'Dutch model of maternity care may not suit Britain'. *BMJ*, 29: 308(6924): 342.

VIL (1999) Verloskundig Vademecum Amstelveen Ziekenfondsraad. http://europe.obgyn.net/nederland/?page=/nederland/richtlijnen/vademecum_eng_statement#Joint%20 Statement. Accessed May 2012.

Walsh, D. and Devane, D. (2012) 'A metasynthesis of midwife-led care'. *Qualitative Health Research*, 22(7): 897–910. http://qhr.sagepub.com/content/22/7/897. Accessed January 2013.

Warren, C. (1994) 'Insurance – Why single out the independent midwife?' *Modern Midwife*, 4(4): 32–3.

WHO (2010) *A Global Survey Monitoring Progress in Nursing and Midwifery*. World Health Organization. WHO/HRH/HPN/10.4 http://www.who.int/hrh/resources/survey/en/index.html. Accessed January 2013.

WHO/ICM/FIGO (2005) 'International definition of the midwife'. World Health Organization/International Confederation of Midwives/International Federation of Gynecology and Obstetrics (WHO/ICM/FIGO). Geneva: WHO.

Worth, J. (2007) *Call the Midwife A true Story of the East End in the 1950s*. London: Phoenix.

PART 1

The scope of midwifery

1

STUDYING MIDWIFERY

Kirsty Darroch and Valerie Fleming

Expectations versus reality

I consider my expectations of midwifery to have been relatively realistic. After all, I had at least some grasp of what the role of the midwife entailed, as it was largely down to the midwifery care I received during my own childbearing experiences that cemented my decision to become a midwife.

My expectations prior to commencing were simple: a caring role that would be predominantly rewarding and fulfilling while undoubtedly being both physically and emotionally demanding. I did not picture midwifery as cute fluffy babies all wrapped in pink or blue while we pranced about looking glamorous! But nor did I anticipate the often backbreaking emotional rollercoaster and almost conveyor belt-like births, liberally scattered with intervention, that were encountered all too frequently in the busy inner-city hospital setting. I merely aspired to provide women with meaningful support, empower them to birth naturally, and as recommended in Midwifery 2020 (2010), promote midwifery-led care and normality in birth.

The reality initially caused me to feel slightly disillusioned and I found myself questioning the wisdom of my career leap. I had after all anticipated a little more evidence of 'normality' and the 'with-woman' ethos of midwifery but much of what I observed was medicalisation, intervention and midwives under immense pressure from an ever-increasing workload fraught with challenges of many kinds. However, as time marched on, my confidence and competence increased and I reflected on practice and began shaping myself into the midwife I had sought to become. I made the reality work for me: I clung on during the rollercoaster ride and have stepped off feeling exhilarated, satisfied and fulfilled.

Embarking on the journey

As it was for me, the commencement of an undergraduate or pre-registration midwifery programme may be the first experience of university and hospital systems for many students (Green & Baird 2009) and as such, has the capacity to rouse mixed emotions. As a direct-entry midwifery student, I had absolutely no previous nursing or medical experience whatsoever and had only attended college many years ago as a teenager! So I can clearly recall feeling simultaneously terrified and desperately excited upon entering the classroom on day one of this life-changing journey. However, making that leap into new and previously unknown territory often instills a huge sense of achievement, which continues to drive the learner forward and maintains motivation, thus facilitating a positive learning experience.

As the International Confederation of Midwives (2010) states, the purpose of midwifery education is to create safe, effective practitioners who will provide care of the highest possible standard to women and their families. So, by necessity, midwifery is taught and thereby learned through a combination of theory (academic learning) and practice (clinical learning). As stipulated by the European Union, the balance of theory to practice must consist of 'no less than 50 per cent practice and no less than 40 per cent theory' (Nursing and Midwifery Council 2009) and may employ a variety of learning and teaching strategies, including simulation.

The curriculum for pre-registration midwifery education is determined by Nursing and Midwifery Council (2009) standards and midwife teachers within a university setting provide the academic theory. With many institutions offering the programme it is inevitable that there will be variances in its delivery, but the European Union Directive 2005/36/EC states clear outcomes incorporating general and specific subjects as well as issues to be covered in the clinical setting. All member states are required to adhere to this and consequently all education programmes contain some degree of similarity.

Rather than focus wholly on the curriculum and format of midwifery education, we now consider some of the more salient points throughout the journey. Along the route there are numerous experiences that are immeasurably valuable both on a personal level and also as an overall positive aspect of midwifery training. For example, the overwhelming awe and wonder when I first assisted a woman to give birth to her baby and the immense privilege of being a guest at what is undoubtedly one of a woman's or couple's most intimate moments will remain two of my abiding memories.

Other than relating my own reasons for becoming a midwife and points along the ensuing journey, several positive curriculum-based areas are also worth touching upon. One such aspect is a midwifery student's supernumerary status. Often regarded as a 'bonus' in the clinical setting where staff shortages abound, this can afford the student the luxury of spending more meaningful time with women in their care who may well be at an emotionally vulnerable stage. As there are fewer demands on the student's time, in some instances rapport and trust may be built readily, whereas, hampered by time constraints and staff shortages, qualified midwives in busy hospitals can sometimes do little more than nod to 'luxuries' such as relationship building whilst carrying out safe, efficient and effective care. As a result, women generally find care provided by students to be beneficial. Snow (2010) studied women's perceptions of care provided by midwifery students, and observed that participants found emotional support was provided through the student's continuous presence, positive and helpful attitude, facilitation of maternal trust and the sharing of a sense of 'mutual newness'. The same study also considers the value of midwifery students acting as 'companions' and raises it as a gentle reminder to all midwives of the true meaning of with woman.

Another positive aspect for me was a caseloading assignment undertaken during the second year of my studies, which was both rewarding and daunting in equal measure! Simply put, this means the student (with predominantly indirect mentor supervision) was responsible for booking up to three women for maternity care and ultimately following them throughout their entire pregnancy and childbearing continuum; thus antenatal, intra-partum and postnatal periods. My particular mentor had great faith in my abilities (she had mentored me on previous occasions) and was more than happy to let me take the lead, knowing that I would work within my own limitations and would approach her or another member of the team if I had any concerns. Her belief in me boosted my confidence and allowed the realisation to dawn that in fact, I knew more than I gave myself credit for. Student caseloading is not a new phenomenon. Bournemouth University pioneered it in 1996, claiming holistic, woman-centred care as central to their pre-registration midwifery education and integral to this was caseloading. Current United Kingdom Standards for Pre-registration Midwifery Education (NMC 2009) also state that students should be afforded the opportunity to practise continuity of care through caseloading, and indeed Lewis *et al.* (2008) describe it as pivotal in promoting women's choice and control. So, upon concluding my assignment, I was somewhat amazed to discover that I had indeed considered, planned and provided safe and effective midwifery care to these women and was rewarded by very positive feedback from them as well as my mentor, and a great sense of satisfaction.

Academically, problem-based learning (PBL) is thought to improve students' knowledge of 'real life' situations by using problem-solving activities and learning to work within teams. PBL was advocated almost two decades ago by the World Health Organization (1993) and is still a popular teaching tool today. Initially, due to ignorance of the benefits on my part, I dismissed PBL as lecturers shirking their teaching duties and delighting in seeing us spend our days off chained to the library desk! However, as time wore on, I found these frequent exercises to be hugely beneficial to me in many ways and understood their relevance in our education. They required us to research, read and ultimately give presentations on topics that we had until then known very little about, which generally worked out well unless someone on the team didn't fully share the workload. By pushing me out of my comfort zone, PBL forced me to face one of my biggest personal fears – standing in front of a roomful of people and speaking to them without sounding completely idiotic. Not only did I conquer my fear, but I consistently received extremely complimentary feedback from my lecturers by the latter period of my studies.

So what of the difficulties encountered during midwifery training? I experienced the odd horrendous shift or two; the essay that I just couldn't make any headway with; or the feeling that my brain may have exploded if I crammed any more into it. However, one recurring theme throughout much of the literature points to students' lack of self-belief or self-confidence in their own skills and abilities; feeling insufficiently prepared for practice; lacking emotional strength and experiencing fear or anxiety that they will not meet the expectations of other midwives and therefore not be successful as an autonomous, accountable practitioner. Much research is available providing more detail on this subject; however, the focus of this chapter is more the educational journey and experience of becoming a midwife and the preparedness that results: confidence (or the lack of) is but one component within the structure. It is however worth touching on. Skirton *et al.* (2011) found confidence in the newly qualified midwife to be a significant feature in their study and claim that while newly qualified midwives are often able to cope with many challenging clinical situations in a safe manner, they frequently report a lack of confidence in their own abilities. The feelings of one newly qualified midwife in particular can be empathised with. Initially, when discussing her newfound responsibility, she alluded to concerns that she lacked ability, which in turn negatively impacted on her confidence. However, upon exploration of these feelings she concluded that rather than any lack of competence or knowledge, ergo ability, it was more likely to be simply a lack of confidence, which should grow through time and with experience.

Licqurish and Seibold (2007) carried out a study using grounded theory and gathered data from eight final-year Australian midwifery students using in-depth interviews to ascertain the impact of the mentor/preceptor on the students' learning and development. Although there were limitations due to a small sample size and little feedback from mentors, the findings – specifically those relating to confidence – are nonetheless very insightful. It was found that midwife mentors who were considered 'helpful' benefited the student by being supportive, allowing hands-on practice and mistakes, shared their knowledge, were motivated and encouraged the students to take responsibility, make decisions and develop new skills. Students cited being given opportunities for responsibility for care and hands-on learning as key factors in developing their confidence and competence. The flip side to this was the 'unhelpful' preceptor who was generally unsupportive, took over care, failed to provide learning opportunities – particularly hands-on learning – for the student and were inconsistent with advice and practice and therefore poor role models. These partnerships left students feeling that they learned very little and as a result seriously lacked confidence: one student claims her mentor 'crushed' her confidence to the point where she felt unable to continue.

Prevost (2011), a final-year midwifery student, concluded in her appraisal of mentorship provision that if the quality of clinical education is compromised – whether through mentor apathy at having to teach, lack of incentive, time constraints, demands of the job or lack of commitment – the effectiveness of the clinical education becomes dubious. She surmises that if factors such as these continue to affect the quality of mentorship, so the quality of future midwives may suffer. I consider myself to have been extremely fortunate with most mentors allocated to me. One in particular stands out as having been a godsend when it came to the matter of my confidence. She knew I possessed all the qualities and attributes of a good midwife – she believed in me when I didn't believe in myself – and so she pushed me out of my comfort zone at times, allowed me innumerable questions and doubts and empowered me to go out there feeling sure of myself and safe. I therefore strongly agree with Evans and Choucri (2012) who found excellent mentorship in the clinical area as being key in enabling this transition from student to newly qualified midwife to be smooth.

Conflicting demands

Whilst anecdotal, an article written by Pallett (2009) manages to encapsulate some of the myriad facets to midwifery training. As a final-year midwifery student she observes that it is often any combination of terrifying, hilarious or exhausting and frequently very rewarding. She goes on to make reference to the juggling of assignments and academic deadlines – of which it seems there are a never-ending stream – and the struggle we often encounter in retaining a semblance of 'normality' in the non-midwifery side of our lives. A difficult task indeed with partners, children and families often making sacrifices to enable us to keep going and be there to talk us round in our darker hours.

There are undoubtedly instances throughout every midwife's training where she doubts whether or not she will ever survive long enough to become a fully-fledged midwife. Much of this can be attributed to the somewhat demanding academic timetable and associated deadlines, some to the predominantly unsocial shift patterns and of course the fact that the two often clash, with academic deadlines still requiring to be met regardless of how many twelve-hour night shifts we might have just ploughed through!

> Learners are also caught between the two worlds of clinical practice and academia, continually having to adapt in order to belong to these worlds and also cope with the significant differences between them.
>
> *(Snow 2010)*

However, with enough forward planning and by utilising good time-management skills, such deadlines should be less of an issue – much of midwifery is after all a massive exercise in time-management and prioritisation.

In relation to some of the academic teaching, the question 'what does this have to do with becoming a midwife?' inevitably arose now and again. Why the need for – what felt at times like – an excess of classroom-based hours and intense afternoons spent immersed in books, journals and research articles? However, on nearing the end of my training, I found myself able to reflect upon the pre-registration midwifery programme as a whole and more specifically the theory-to-practice ratio.

Realisation finally dawned that it all forms part of our essential learning as midwives, enabling us to build up a knowledge base that aids us in recognising normality. For, without recognition of normality, how would we recognise deviations from it? The other 'part' is, of course, our clinical experience, where we learn to apply theory to practice and develop a skill set fundamental to midwifery practice.

A prospective longitudinal qualitative study undertaken by Skirton et al. (2011) explored whether, upon completion of the pre-registration midwifery programme, newly qualified midwives in the UK were sufficiently prepared and competent for practice. They gathered data from newly qualified midwives within the initial 6 months of their first midwifery post. Amongst their findings was the existence of a close, symbiotic inter-relationship between the teaching of knowledge and practical experience, indicating that the two do indeed go hand in hand. One new midwife articulated this relationship between theoretical knowledge and practical experience as only becoming apparent upon qualifying, where it began to 'make sense', and allowed understanding of both the purpose and importance of the two aspects. Similarly, in their article considering the transition from student to newly qualified midwife, Evans and Choucri (2012) highlight that emotional intelligence and a fine attitude are no replacement for competence and that it is indeed the balance of skills that is crucial in the delivery of safe, holistic midwifery care.

McIntosh et al. (2012) make reference to the 'preparedness' dilemma of midwifery students as stemming primarily from two camps: one housing the risk-averse National Health Service and professional regulatory bodies while the other contains the university beliefs of education being negotiable and revisable. Their belief is that students are not in fact caught in a theory–practice gap, but instead trapped between two powerful contributors in the application of knowledge.

Preparedness/transition

> By developing personally, professionally and educationally, a student midwife has arrived at a place of transition where she will cross over from having student status to being a fully registered midwife in her own right.
>
> *(Evans & Choucri 2012)*

When the issue of preparedness for practice is raised, it is worth considering Pallett's (2009) observations. She found it to be that midwifery students are often criticised the most by other midwives, some of whom regard us as exiting our training with insufficient clinical practice, inadequate training, not enough 'numbers' and generally considering us unprepared for practice. Further to this, Pallett suggests that our critics would be better placed supporting us to achieve the level of skill required to provide safe, evidence-based, individualised and woman-centred care and therefore enabling us to feel a deeper sense of preparedness. But then, mentoring and the attitudes of other midwives is a whole other topic!

With the exception of community placements and one short week spent with the home birth team, all clinical placements I completed were hospital-based and more to the point single-site. By this I refer to the fact that all clinical training over the course of my three years was undertaken at just one hospital. So now, on completion of my midwifery training, I have taken time to reflect on whether or not I have been trained as a flexible and adaptable midwife or more as a midwife suited only to working in an inner-city hospital. How well prepared am I for working in, for example, a rural midwifery post? Am I prepared enough for practising midwifery in another country? Or even for that matter, in another setting within the same country?

Van der Putten (2008) cites Kramer's (1974) findings on the phenomenon known as 'reality shock'. Kramer refers to 'specific shock-like reactions' from newly qualified nurses who entered into a position for which they considered themselves prepared, only to discover they were not. A sudden increase in responsibility along with their newfound accountability found many feeling stressed and unprepared which led to feelings of anxiety and trepidation. One newly qualified midwife in van der Putten's study describes being 'delighted' to have qualified but also uses words such as 'nerve-wracking', 'daunting' and 'terrified' on describing her first shift as a newly qualified midwife on labour ward.

Although undertaken at a single university in Victoria, Australia, Licqurish and Seibold (2012) found midwifery students were generally considered competent for practice upon completion of their studies. However, some participants reported feeling inhibited by the medical dominance within the clinical area in which they were placed as well as a lack of clinical hours allocated in which to achieve competencies and personal learning objectives. The majority of hospitals that students were assigned to did not support autonomous practice, nor did they offer much in the way of continuity of care, highlighting a significant theory–practice gap. Students reported vast differences between what was detailed in their professional competencies against the reality of midwifery practice 'in the system' and this is further reiterated in van der Putten's (2008) study where findings illustrate discrepancies between that taught in the academic environment and how care is provided in the clinical area.

There is a wealth of literature surrounding the issue of the theory–practice gap but this can only be touched upon here. McIntosh et al. (2012) recognise that for some time now, the spotlight has been on this gap in clinical education and concerns have been voiced by many that newly qualified midwives are unprepared for the realities of clinical practice (Donovan 2008; Holland et al. 2010). McIntosh et al. (2012) have recently published an excellent in-depth analysis of the experience of becoming a midwife, within which are considerable column inches devoted to how we learn and the fact that it is impossible to 'know it all'. The need to be able to respond to the unknown will always be present – some students accepted that even midwives of many years' experience don't know everything. The study also highlights that there is a blurring of the boundaries between what constitutes preparedness and knowing it all; knowledge sometimes being mistaken for preparedness.

Regardless of how prepared or unprepared any newly qualified midwife may be for the big wide world of midwifery, the journey will have been nothing less than remarkable. Hopefully it will be memorable for primarily positive reasons, although a few not-so-positive encounters will invariably find their way into the overall mix. What is important is that all experiences are viewed as learning opportunities, and whether good or bad these enrich our knowledge. This anonymous quote sums up beautifully how I feel about my midwifery training:

> Every day may not be good, but there's something good in every day.
>
> *(Author unknown)*

Personally, it sometimes astounds me that I came through this relatively unscathed!

So, upon entering my first job as a newly qualified midwife I must now look to the future. In order to ensure my continued professional development through life-long learning I shall routinely consider my learning needs and plan how best to take them forward.

NHS Education Scotland (2009), within their document 'Towards 2020: Consensus Statement', which focuses on practice learning, claim that as a registered midwife (newly qualified or not),

> Learning is an ongoing process that is supported and developed through interaction and therapeutic relationships. The quality of practice learning experiences is improved through individual learners responding to feedback from service users and those who support them.
>
> *(NHS Education Scotland 2009)*

Which once again reiterates that ongoing learning is our own responsibility and we must reflect and also consider feedback from others when identifying our own learning requirements.

Continuing education for midwives

Kirsty's account of her education shows that a sound preparation was in place to undertake the complex role of the midwife in present times. However, midwifery education does not end with the gaining of the qualification. Indeed the UK has in place a robust requirement for continuing education by all midwives comprising 450 hours of registered practice and 35 hours of learning activity (Continuing Professional Development) in the previous three years (NMC 2012). Similar conditions exist in other countries; with Switzerland, for example, while not legislating, including generous continuing education time in continuing education for midwives. New Zealand has even more stringent requirements with a recertification programme for all midwives having been in place since 2007 (te Tatau o te Whare Kahu 2012).

Choosing an educational activity

It is relatively unlikely that a midwife, at the point of qualification, will know exactly the direction her career is going to take and remain committed to that direction for up to a further 40–50 years. In my own case my initial ambition was to be a nurse (for which I needed the midwifery qualification) on a cruise ship. During my midwifery education programme that changed to wanting to be a 'ward sister' in the labour ward and in the next few years it was revised many times. However, I never imagined that when I qualified in 1979 I would become a senior adviser in the World Health Organization or a professor of midwifery in two countries. For me, the more I learned the more I have to learn and I can honestly say that none of my formal learning has been wasted even though at times I questioned its value!

Further education, unlike the initial programme, allows midwives the freedom to choose subjects that are relevant to their own practice, or perhaps embrace an area into which they would like to move. Such courses are also likely to incur a charge so it makes sense that potential participants find out as much as they can in advance to ensure that their own aims are compatible with those of the course.

In-service education

Most employers will offer midwives in-house-run courses that are often free of charge and embrace policy and practice issues that are necessary for employees to master. There is no question of the relevance of these courses, as they are mostly necessary for the midwife to be able to function in her role, and midwives undertaking these may find it necessary to attend on more than one occasion as it is vital to be fully competent before undertaking the task in question. Examples of such courses are related to the moving and handling of patients, the use of specialised equipment and emergency procedures.

Other courses offered by the employing institution may embrace areas that are broader than simply midwifery but afford the opportunity for midwives to undertake these with other health professionals and so to broaden their outlook on a particular area of concern or get to know her colleagues in other departments. Such programmes, while likely to be subject to a charge, often are subsidised by the employer or an external agency and generally represent good value for money. An area that might be embraced in such a short course is that of inter-cultural care which is especially relevant where midwives should be providing care for women from cultural or ethnic backgrounds with which they are not familiar.

Conferences

Each year there are many conferences lasting one or more days. At first the choice may seem bewildering with many of them appearing attractive to the midwife who is looking for fresh information to supplement her basic education. Some conferences are for midwives, others for multidisciplinary groups, or for consumers and midwives; some are billed as national and yet others international. Some offer credit points to certain occupational groups; all cost money, yet costs do not seem to be related to content.

Making a choice thus is not easy. However, taking part in conferences is a good way to network and share common interests and concerns. It is therefore worthwhile taking the time before registering for conferences to work out a budget, seek appropriate conferences and after scanning them carefully, discussing them with colleagues who may previously have attended. Key questions to ask are, 'Who are the keynote speakers?', 'How do the parallel sessions function?' (e.g. is it possible to move from room to room within groups of sessions; how many participants do the rooms hold; is it necessary to register for each session in advance?), 'What extra costs are involved?' (e.g. for special workshops or evening entertainment), 'Is my employer prepared to give me the time or must I use my annual leave?', 'How long will it take me to reach the venue?'

Sometimes employers will now only allow conference attendance in work time if a presentation is being made. This takes a lot of courage but is a worthwhile exercise as it will promote discussion on a topic of personal interest. To submit an abstract for presentation it is necessary not only to have done the necessary background work on the subject, but also to follow the conference committee's guidelines closely. If anything is ambiguous, an email should be sent to the conference organisers requesting clarification. The abstract will be reviewed by a committee and applicants notified in plenty of time to prepare the presentations. All presentations should be carefully prepared and not overloaded with slides. Key information only should be on the slides and the oral presentation built up around these. Ideally a presentation should not be read from a paper but nerves may necessitate this on the first few occasions. The discussion by participants can then turn the presentation into a paper for a journal.

University programmes

Like Kirsty, many midwives' basic education is now undertaken at a university. However, in many countries this is still not possible. Some will offer a top-up programme to degree level, while other midwives wishing to study academically may have to choose programmes in other disciplines.

Of course for many newly qualified midwives the thought of more study is the last thing they want to do. Instead all they want to do is practise their profession. This is understandable, but as mentioned earlier in this chapter, there is a requirement for midwives to continue their education in order to maintain their competence. For some (further) university study will be the answer.

As with other forms of continuing education, what kind of programme is chosen is dependent on availability and cost. However, the midwife also needs to take into consideration expected workload. It may be that she decides on one module which requires three hours attendance per week. However, behind this requirement are many hours of private study and these must be factored in. While everyone works at an individual pace, as a general rule one European credit point (ECTS) is considered approximately 25 hours of study. A module worth 10 ECTS therefore will incur about 250 hours of expected student effort.

Another choice to make is whether to undertake a programme that is offered by face-to-face teaching or whether to undertake distance education programmes (usually by on-line study). A module should take the same amount of time to complete regardless of its mode of teaching, thus the choice is dependent on the student's individual preferences and circumstances. It can sometimes be easier to be motivated when there is a requirement to turn up at a given time each week or when there is an option to work with fellow students in small groups. However, with videoconferencing technology, this is now also possible worldwide, thereby paving the way for rich international exchanging of views.

University study as a qualified midwife is a good opportunity to combine work experience with academic development and there is an array of programmes available in the English-speaking countries and also some others such as Germany and Scandinavia at various levels from Bachelor's to Doctoral degrees.

Continuing education and promoted posts in the profession

Some posts such as consultant midwives in the UK will be linked to specific academic education requirements but many others are not. However, the midwife who can demonstrate that she has gained from her further education rather than doing it because it is obligatory is likely to be considered more favourably for promoted posts.

Conclusion

As a career, midwifery can be both challenging and rewarding, and in order for midwives to remain capable of providing safe, evidence-based practice, it is crucial that we keep abreast of the very latest knowledge and research. Although midwifery education provides a sound basis for practice, it will continually require updating due to the dynamic nature of midwifery. Continued education enables the integration of new ideas as well as the generation and development of these from practice. Therefore, so long as a midwife remains in practice, continuing education must remain a priority – a conduit to enable the provision of excellent care.

References

Donovan, P. (2008) 'Confidence in newly qualified midwives'. *British Journal of Midwifery* 16(8): 510–14. Available at: https://www.intermid.co.uk/cgi-bin/go.pl/library/article.cgi?uid=30784;article=BJM_16_8_510_514

Evans, S. and Choucri, L. (2012) 'Transitioning from a student to a midwife: A first-hand account'. *British Journal of Midwifery* 20(3): 211–214. Available at: http://www.intermid.co.uk/cgi-bin/go.pl/library/article.cgi?uid=89968;article=BJM_20_3_211_214

Green, S. and Baird, K. (2009) 'An exploratory, comparative study investigating attrition and retention of student midwives'. *Midwifery* 25: 79–87. Available at: http://www.science direct.com/science/article/pii/S0266613807001155

Holland, K., Roxburgh, M., Johnson, M., Topping, K., Watson, R., Lauder, W. *et al.* (2010) 'Fitness for practice in nursing and midwifery education in Scotland, United Kingdom'. *Journal of Clinical Nursing* 19(3–4): 461–69. Available at: http://onlinelibrary.wiley.com/doi/10.1111/j.1365-2702.2009.03056.x/abstract;jsessionid=E5B3D8E75C57B6B5EDD35BE5546F414C.d04t02

International Confederation of Midwives (2010) 'Global standards for midwifery education'. Available at: http://www.internationalmidwives.org/Documentation/ICMGlobalStandardsCompetenciesandTools/GlobalStandardsEnglish/tabid/980/Default.aspx

Lewis, P., Fry, J. and Rawnson, S. (2008) 'Student midwife caseloading – a new approach to midwifery education'. *British Journal of Midwifery* 16(8): 499–502. Available at: http://www.intermid.co.uk/cgi-bin/go.pl/library/article.cgi?uid=30782;article=BJM_16_8_499_502;format=pdf

Licqurish, S. and Seibold, C. (2012) '"Chasing the numbers": Australian Bachelor of Midwifery students' experiences of achieving midwifery practice requirements for registration'. *Midwifery* 29(6): 661–7. Available at: http://www.sciencedirect.com/science/article/pii/S0266613812001064

Licqurish, S. and Seibold, C. (2007) 'Bachelor of Midwifery students' experiences of achieving competencies: The role of the midwife preceptor'. *Midwifery* 24(4): 480–89. Available at: http://www.sciencedirect.com/science/article/pii/S0266613807000745

McIntosh, T., Fraser, D.M., Stephen, N. and Avis, M. (2012) 'Final year students' perceptions of learning to be a midwife in six British universities'. *Nurse Education Today* 33(10): 1179–83. Available at: http://www.sciencedirect.com/science/article/pii/S0260691712001724

Midwifery 2020 (2010) *Core role of the midwife workstream final report*. Available at: http://www.midwifery2020.org/Core%20and%20Developing%20Role%20of%20the%20Midwife/index.asp

NHS Education Scotland (2009) *Clinical Education Career Framework*. Edinburgh: NES Scotland.

Nursing and Midwifery Council (NMC), (2009) *Standards for Pre-Registration Midwifery Education*. Available at: http://www.nmc-uk.org/Documents/NMC-Publications/nmcStandardsforPre_RegistrationMidwiferyEducation.pdf

Nursing and Midwifery Council (NMC) (2012) *Midwives Rules and Standards*. Available at: http://www.nmc-uk.org/Documents/NMC-Publications/Midwives%20Rules%20and%20Standards%202012.pdf

Pallett, S. (2009) 'Training, what training?' *Birthspirit Midwifery*, 1: 55.

Prevost, M. (2011) 'Mentorship: an appraisal from a student midwife's perspective'. *MIDIRS Midwifery Digest*, 21(3): 292–96.

Skirton, H., Stephen, N., Doris, F., Cooper, M., Avis, M. and Fraser, D.M. (2011) 'Preparedness of newly qualified midwives to deliver clinical care: An evaluation of pre-registration midwifery education through an analysis of key events'. *Midwifery* 28(5): 660–66. Available at: http://www.sciencedirect.com/science/article/pii/S0266613811001215

Snow, S. (2010) '"Mutual newness": mothers' experiences of student midwives'. *British Journal of Midwifery* 18(1): 38–41. Available at: http://www.intermid.co.uk/cgi-bin/go.pl/library/article.cgi?uid=45814;article=BJM_18_1_38_41

te Tatau o te Whare Kahu (2012) 'Standards for recertification of midwives.' Available at: http://www.midwiferycouncil.health.nz/education/

Unknown author, http://dailypositivequotes.com/quotes/every-day-may-not-be-good-but-there-is-something-good-in-everyday

van der Putten, D. (2008) 'The lived experience of newly qualified midwives: a qualitative study'. *British Journal of Midwifery* 16(6): 348–58. Available at: http://www.interm id.co.uk/cgi-bin/go.pl/library/article.cgi?uid=29592;article=BJM_16_6_348_358

World Health Organization (1993) *Increasing the Relevance of Education for Health Professionals: Report of a WHO Study Group on Problem-Solving Education for the Health Professions.* WHO, Geneva. Available at: http://www.sciencedirect.com/science/article/pii/S01688510949 00655.

Commentary

Kirsty presents an admirably balanced, yet realistic, picture of the experience of a 'mature' midwifery student, which represents the experience of a gratifyingly increasing proportion of midwifery students. She recounts insightfully the highs and lows of her midwifery programme without falling in to the all too common trap of blaming individuals for what may be shortcomings in the system of midwifery education. Valerie's follow-on account of continuing professional development reminds us of the mind-boggling variety of opportunities to enable the midwife to maintain and enhance her expertise.

Together, these two views of different aspects of midwifery education really serve to bring home both the depth and the breadth of the knowledge base on which midwifery is built. It may be, though, that we should accept more explicitly that this knowledge base includes some other, less tangible, forms of knowledge. As well as the fundamental theoretical knowledge and other knowledge derived from occupational and personal experience, including many midwives' personal childbearing experience, we may need to contemplate others. These include the less substantial areas such as some types of instinct and also what may be termed 'gut feelings'. In this way, a wide variety of 'knowledges', some of which may be largely subjective (Belenky *et al.* 1997), would be given the recognition which they deserve.

Reference

Belenky, M.F., Clinchy, B.M., Goldberger, N.R. and Tarule, J.M. (1997) *Women's Ways of Knowing: The Development of Self, Voice, and Mind.* New York: Basic Books.

2

MIDWIFERY CARE IN THE COMMUNITY DURING THE WOMAN'S PREGNANCY

Yvonne Fontein

VIGNETTE

'Pregnant, but not happy', that's how I felt. After all these years I was finally pregnant but I did not feel happy and I was scared to tell anyone. That was until today, when meeting my midwife changed my feelings somehow. I was very apprehensive to go and see her and did not plan to share my feelings with her. But somehow she managed to ask all the right questions, to recognise my worries and to give me the feeling that I am actually allowed feeling this. When she and I listened to the baby's heartbeat it made me realise there is really a baby growing in me. Although I am glad we still have a long way to go before this baby will arrive, somehow I think I will be able to get through this and to start enjoying what is ahead of me, and I am sure there is someone out there to look after me and this baby.

Stories such as this made me realise that pregnancy is a major event in the life of a woman and her family and represents a journey to motherhood. How to become a caring, safe and considerate midwife to accompany the woman's journey is influenced by the fact that every woman is unique, each pregnancy is an original journey and every experience is special. There appears to be no such thing as an average woman in an ordinary community needing routine care. This kindled my interest in becoming a midwife.

The woman's pregnancy and the midwife

There are ideas and philosophies that form the foundations of how the midwife takes care of a woman during her pregnancy – known as antenatal care. Although midwives have been doing this for centuries, these ideas are given such names as holistic midwifery, woman-centred care, partnership and assessment of well-being. These ideas and philosophies need some explanation to understand them and how a midwife can use them to underpin her work while caring for pregnant women, and how they are incorporated and experienced by the midwife on a day-to-day basis.

Holistic midwifery

Pregnancy is represented by the physical changes in the woman's body. However, it also involves other dimensions of the woman, such as her mind or emotions. One of these dimensions can influence the other; if a woman is feeling very unhappy, this can have an effect on her physical condition in pregnancy, as anxieties and worries can cause an imbalance in a pregnant woman's physical health. The woman's relationship with her partner, family circumstances, housing, worries about motherhood, work and finances are examples that can influence a woman's health and can, for example, affect blood pressure or cause morning sickness (Kurki *et al.* 2000; Buckwalter and Simpson 2002; Swallow *et al.* 2004). A woman can experience feelings of guilt towards her unborn baby when she smokes, or her altering body image, as a result of pregnancy, can make a woman feel unattractive and cause feelings of depression. As these are very normal day-to-day aspects of pregnancy, this illustrates that pregnancy is not just a physical experience that can be separated from the woman as a whole.

To address the full context of the woman and her pregnancy as a total integrated concept is called holistic midwifery (Walsh and Steen 2007). Taking into account the whole concept of the woman's emotional, psychological, social, physical, cultural, spiritual needs and expectations and their relationship makes a midwife a holistic midwife.

Woman-centred care

Pregnancy is an experience in a woman's life that has a different value or meaning to every individual woman. When a woman presents herself for her first antenatal visit, the midwife has to appreciate that a woman brings in her experiences of the past, her present needs and her expectations and hopes for the future. Although it is the element and presence of pregnancy itself that brings the woman into contact with the midwife, the woman also brings with her this total package of herself, her being and the community she is part of. Recognising, acknowledging and respecting the individual woman and her unique needs, ideas, thoughts, emotions, expectations and wishes about pregnancy, motherhood and childbirth related issues, is known as woman-centred care, in other words, the woman and her unborn baby come first (Leap and Homer 2002).

Partnership

The concept of working in partnership with a woman is an important contributing factor for the midwife to achieve woman-centred care.

This means a process of teamwork between a woman, her partner or significant others and the midwife, working towards a shared goal, which can entail all sorts of issues such as place of birth and so on – in general, a healthy pregnancy and a healthy baby. Partnership is characterised by an exchange of the midwife's knowledge and expertise and the woman's expectations, needs, anxieties and experiences. The midwife contributes her or his knowledge and professional experience and the woman brings her package of personal needs, wishes, questions, uncertainties or anxieties. The midwife has to give sound information to a woman to offer her realistic choices in relation to topics such as antenatal tests, but also to make her aware of the choices available. Therefore, it is an exchange of information between the midwife and the woman; the midwife has the responsibility to inform a woman about her options and choices, while the woman has to inform the midwife of her needs in order to address them.

This implies that both the woman and the midwife contribute to the relationship they have, which is focused on the pregnancy and the journey into motherhood. The fact that both the woman and the midwife are contributing to the childbirth experience from a different angle and background enhances the professional role and responsibility of the midwife as well as the personal part the woman plays in this joint adventure of childbirth.

Day-to-day practice

The midwife's work is a fusion of knowledge and competencies and it is a composite of a variety of skills that are incorporated into day-to-day practice. Practical skills, such as record keeping, are utilised during antenatal visits alongside a range of counselling and communication skills, all performed with a professional attitude and knowledge. On the one hand, assessing well-being is the main focus of antenatal care, but, on the other hand, antenatal care comprises immense variety and diversity. All skills are applied in a day's work during which the midwife meets pregnant women, assesses their pregnancies and well-being, provides the necessary information, listens to their worries and thoughts, tries to address their needs, supports them in making choices, documents findings, makes appointments for future visits, refers women to other appropriate health professionals and provides education. All of these issues are addressed when a single antenatal visit is often restricted to 10 minutes. Antenatal care is dynamic and the midwife will hardly experience a dull moment when involved with women and their families.

VIGNETTE

My day . . .

It is late afternoon when I finish my antenatal clinic of that day. While I am clearing up I reflected on my day. The clinic has started at 9.00 AM but immediately went different from how I had planned it. The practice assistant of the GP surgery, where my antenatal clinic of that day is located, invited me in her office to discuss something. It was about Shana, a young girl pregnant with her third child, currently using methadone. She had not picked up her methadone for a couple of days and the practice assistant was worried. In response to her worries I tried to phone Shana but there was no reply. I told the practice assistant that I would visit Shana after my clinic that afternoon as I had another home visit planned anyway. One more would not do me any harm. I was ready to start but the first client was late for her booking appointment and therefore I started later than planned. A booking visit lasts 30 minutes but there are so many things to discuss (past medical history, previous pregnancies and births, counselling about prenatal tests, discussing things like domestic violence, smoking and drinking behaviour) and to do (taking blood pressure, taking bloods, testing urine, weighing) that it is hard to get everything done in those 30 minutes. Luckily the woman was very healthy and felt fine, was happy to be pregnant and declined information about prenatal testing. So, although I was late it was not too bad. Just when I thought I was getting on schedule again, Theresa arrived. She was pregnant with her second child and was now in the third trimester of pregnancy; she still had six weeks to go before her due date. Approaching the end of pregnancy had made her realise that the birth was getting nearer, something she previously did not want to discuss as she had experienced the birth of her first child as traumatic. Now she was ready to talk. But was I? Knowing I still had a lot of women to see that morning and being aware that Shana was on my agenda later that day, I listened to Theresa's story and her fears and worries while I was checking her blood pressure, growth of the baby, the foetal heart rate and making notes. I suggested to Theresa to make a birth plan to outline her expectations, which is a written plan where she can record her personal ideas and wishes and needs about the forthcoming birth (such as positioning during birth, pain relief, and the role of her partner). She was quite upset while she talked. I made a note about her feelings in relation to the birth and my suggestion about the birth plan in her records, so my colleague who would see Theresa for the next appointment could hopefully discuss this with Theresa more thoroughly. I knew I had only ten minutes for Theresa, as that is all the time we have for an antenatal visit, but spotted Deidre's name while I quickly glanced in the agenda. She was scheduled for the next appointment. For Deidre, pregnancy seemed smooth sailing, she was never late, never complained, never wanted to discuss anything in particular and always left within five minutes. Giving Theresa more time, I hoped I would get back on schedule again with Deidre. But still I knew I did not have enough time to give Theresa the attention, the support and advice she really needed and of which I knew I could give her, if only I had enough time. Out of the window went my ideas about holistic care, partnership and woman-centred care, things I believed in but which are not always achievable with a busy clinic. I love doing clinics but sometimes it frustrates me; like today. I made a mental note to discuss length of appointment time during the next practice meeting. Why not change an appointment to 15 minutes or even better, into 20? That way we would be able to meet the needs of the women we look after. When Deidre came in, accepting my apology for being late, I immediately saw something was wrong with her. She didn't look well at all. After I had checked her blood pressure, her urine and checked the baby's growth, I was quite concerned. Her blood pressure was too high, there was protein in her urine, the baby seemed not to have grown since her last appointment and she told me she had headaches, stomach pain and she thought the baby did not move as much as before. My alarm bells started ringing. The baby's heartbeat was fine but I told Deidre I was going to phone the hospital immediately as I wanted to have her checked for HELLP syndrome. I explained to Deidre what I suspected and what she could expect in the hospital; I arranged for her husband to come and pick her up to drive to the hospital. After Deidre left I just gave up about my schedule and worked throughout my lunch break, eating my sandwiches in between two appointments. The afternoon clinic went a bit better with just a few hiccoughs: a phone call from the hospital about Deidre letting me know my suspicions had been correct and that she was admitted into the hospital. A woman who needed referral to the physiotherapist because of lower back pain and pelvic pain. A child who thought my doptone, worth €500, was a toy, dropped it on the floor while I was checking his mother's blood pressure. Someone who was going on a holiday needing a letter declaring she was allowed to fly and while I was trying to print it, the printer gave up. But apart from these small issues, it went rather well. After some administrative tasks, I was ready to go and see Shana.

The journey

At the moment a woman finds out that she is pregnant, she envisages her future and what this will be like in 9 months' time. The journey of pregnancy and preparation for motherhood starts at the very beginning of the pregnancy, when a woman attends her first antenatal visit; a midwife is privileged to make the journey of childbirth with a woman and her significant others, to support them, facilitate them in the process and guide them through their journey. However, the period of pregnancy is time-restricted, as it lasts for approximately 40 weeks. Pregnancy is, therefore, a short but intense period leading into motherhood, which in itself is a lifelong event and will eventually integrate into a woman's life as it continues on its path. Although the midwife only participates in a short episode in the woman's journey through life on the whole, it is obvious that he or she has an important role to play in the short but profound time-span of pregnancy and birth. The midwife accompanies the woman and her family, starting at the beginning of pregnancy, aiming to prepare and equip them as best as can be achieved for the journey ahead. This is not a routine job because it impacts on the individual life of a woman, her partner and family, regardless of the outcome of the pregnancy. Every year a child's birthday is going to be celebrated; what the midwife said or did at the time is going to be recalled. My colleague describes it:

> If the voyage of childbirth can be seen as a metaphor of a train journey, the midwife embarks the train in pregnancy and disembarks shortly after the birth of the baby, waves them good-bye and wishes them a further safe and healthy journey.

Midwifery care in the community

A midwife may practise in any setting, including the community and the woman's home (ICM 2005). Although the woman comes first and is the centre of the midwife's care, the woman cannot be separated from the community where she lives. Historically, the midwife always had, and still has, a position and place in the community, serving the childbearing population in a specific area. In the community the midwife can be based in a health centre or a general practitioner's surgery, but the working environment can also include the woman's home.

Midwives work among various populations, each with their specific characteristics, such as level of education or affluence, religion or origin, as well as local health problems and needs or special needs in relation to childbirth. Perceptions of pregnancy and preparation for motherhood are related to their backgrounds and to personal experiences with pregnancy or motherhood. Midwives may be practising within the same country, area or even in the same town, but their care can comprise and focus on completely different aspects. A midwife can be located in a poor area with mixed cultures, including minority groups, where single motherhood, teenage pregnancy and substance abuse frequently occur and where women's own mothers or peers are their informants. Midwifery care here will differ from that of a midwife in an affluent area, with older first-time mothers in stable relationships with established careers, who maybe had to seek medical assistance to become pregnant and who use the internet as their primary source of information. Differences in midwifery care can also be affected and influenced by the level of urbanisation of the community in which the midwife is positioned. The midwife can be based in a city or town where women live near to hospitals and can access maternity services easily. The midwife can also work rurally, where the infrastructure differs from that of an urban area, where women live at a distance from maternity facilities, where pregnancy is a widely accepted aspect of life not needing a lot of fuss or specific attention, and where home birth is the norm. A woman has to be recognised within the wider picture of the society in which she lives, as this influences the woman's perception and experience of the pregnancy and her preparation for motherhood. This needs to be a key aim for the midwife.

When a midwife works in a local community she is familiar with the population in her area, such as levels of affluence and employment, size of local population, housing, cultural diversity, religion, infrastructure such as the accessibility of shops, childcare, health care and emergency services. Statistics in the area of home births and breastfeeding, existing social problems or health issues, for example smoking or teenage pregnancies, are known to the midwife. These facts and figures affect the childbearing population and therefore form the contents of the midwife's parenthood education, which is an important task in antenatal care. The midwife often deals with these issues on an individual level, but also provides this valuable information to groups in the woman's community.

Midwives often refer to women in the community as 'their women', which illustrates the involvement and personal aspect of the relationship between the woman and the midwife, which can have advantages and disadvantages.

VIGNETTE

After living and working in the same area for all these years, it is lovely to see these mums and their children in the streets, knowing I have been involved with all of them and to see them grow up and to remember anecdotes from when they were pregnant. But sometimes I have been worried about women during pregnancy, asking myself if they would be able to look after their children, and involving the health visitor and GP to share my worries. There have been a few moments that I had to involve child protection and had been violently threatened by parents because they were so angry when a child had been taken away from home as a result of my report. There are times that it is impossible to 'just pop into the shops' to get my last minute shopping, as I bump into all these mothers with prams wanting to show their baby, share their stories or ask questions about nappy rash or breastfeeding. This is one of the reasons that my own daughter never wants to come to the shops with me as 'I am always talking to everyone' or 'women always want something from me' or 'why do I always need to look in every pram we pass?'

Working in the woman's home and the health centre

Antenatal care takes place in the health centre as well as in the woman's home, depending on the woman's wishes or circumstances. Circumstances can dictate that a woman may not be able to keep her antenatal appointments, for reasons unknown to the midwife. Inviting or letting the midwife into the home means that the woman does not have to travel to the midwife or have to wait for lengths of time in a surgery's waiting room, which could be full of sick people. It also means, however, being vulnerable when there are visible problems to be observed, such as poverty. Being in the woman's home means that the midwife is the guest and the woman is in control of her environment, while in the health centre, being the midwife's territory, it is the midwife who is in control. In contrast to a clinical health centre or surgery, the personal and individual atmosphere of the woman's home gives the midwife an impression about her home environment and family life, which would have otherwise remained unknown. When a woman is considering a home birth, practicalities are best discussed in the woman's home, where the midwife can assess possibilities for or hindrances to this event.

VIGNETTE

My day continues . . .

I am on way to see Shana and I also have to see Nicola at home. She is 36 weeks pregnant and wants a home birth. When women choose to have a home birth we schedule a home visit around 36 weeks of pregnancy. Not only to discuss the birth and its practicalities when this occurs at home but also to get an impression of how a woman lives. Are there stairs, which would make it impossible to get her downstairs in case of an emergency or referral to the hospital? Are there animals we should know of? I vividly remember a home birth a couple of years ago, before we did home visits, discovering this huge barking dangerous-looking and uncontrollable dog when I arrived at the woman's home for the home birth. It had taken ages for me to get into the house, hearing the woman scream in the house during her contractions while I was standing outside in the snow, waiting for the dog to be shut in a room. Sometimes you have this image of a woman; how she lives, about her partner, etc. Then you visit her at her house and this image can just shatter to pieces, as it is so different than what you expected. For me it can put a woman into a wider perspective, picture her better, and I sometimes find it easier to understand her, having seen what she is talking about. I love doing antenatal home visits; it makes it so much more personal. And you don't have to watch the clock because somebody else will be waiting. When you want to discuss things properly, there is plenty of time at the woman's home and you don't feel the pressure that you have to hurry.

While I am lost in my thoughts, I arrive at Shana's flat. Her flat is located in a less affluent part of the town; a lot of flats in Shana's street are lying empty as the council has decided to demolish this block of flats. When I started to work in the area after graduation, I was too scared to go there on my own, feeling really vulnerable because people shouted really vulgar and horrible things or finding my car being scratched over. Now people in the area know me as 'the' midwife and never bother me. I enter the hallway of Shana's apartment. It is filthy and cans and cigarette stubs lie everywhere. I remember my colleague telling me she once had found a used syringe there. I knock at Shana's front door. After a while her boyfriend opens the door, visibly 'high'. I enter the living room and see Shana lying on the settee, smoking a cigarette. I have been here before and am always drawn to the picture on the wall. It is a lovely picture of a pretty and laughing Shana, obviously taken in the time before she started to use drugs. What a contrast with the girl lying there. This is Shana's third baby over the time-span of four years from three different men. Shana doesn't know if her current boyfriend is the father of this baby. The other children have been taken from her and this baby is going to be taken away from her after it will be born. Shana has threatened to have this baby on her own and run away with it, so I carefully approach her. She has indeed not collected her methadone as she had been using some heroin because she felt so miserable about the baby being taken away. We talk a bit more while I check her blood pressure and the baby, which are fine. What to do now? I tell Shana I am worried about her and I would like her to get her methadone from the surgery. I also say that I think it is better to give her social worker a call. She agrees and I am making the phone call, quickly glancing around in the living room and in the kitchen. It's an absolute mess. There is no carpet on the floor, paint is peeling off the walls and mould stains are on the ceiling. I feel frustrated as there is not a lot I can do, and tell Shana to go the clinic for her check-up. She agrees but I doubt if she will go. Back in the car I phone her GP, the social worker again, and the hospital, to say if Shana were to arrive, could they see her as soon as possible because experience has told me that if she has to wait, she will leave.

What a contrast when I go to see Nicola. Blooming and healthy she opens the door offering me a cup of tea. We discuss her home birth and she shows me the house. She proudly opens the door of the nursery, which is absolutely lovely; everything is ready for this baby to be welcomed in this world.

The midwife in a changing world

The role of the midwife is currently changing as health promotion has expanded the midwife's role (Ross-Davie *et al.* 2006). Although health promotion has always been a part of antenatal care, this was predominantly focused on pregnancy-related issues like breastfeeding, exercise, healthy eating or sexual health. As technology has progressed, this also shows in antenatal care with ultrasound scans, even in 3D and 4D, and possibilities to undertake tests to look for abnormalities. Nowadays midwives have to counsel women about prenatal screening, which means having a test done in early pregnancy to assess the risk of being pregnant of a baby with Down syndrome or some other chromosomal abnormalities. Just envisage that at the beginning of a pregnancy, women and their partners encounter difficult decisions; not only about having this test done but also having to think about possible consequences of the test results. If parents are faced with a result of a high chance of having a baby with Down syndrome, they will have to make a decision to continue with the pregnancy or not. Most women have an ultrasound scan in the middle of pregnancy. Again, this is a moment to check if the baby is healthy. Often women do not realise this and regard a scan as 'fun' or a chance to know if the baby is going to be a boy or a girl. When parents are then suddenly faced with 'bad news', this may come as a total shock. These are difficult topics for parents as well as for the midwife. The midwife may have her own opinion and view but must not express this to parents, as she must not influence parents in their decision. The task of the midwife is to inform them as best as possible, based on sound evidence. Often this means logic and rationale versus emotions.

Midwives also have to ask women very personal questions about their lives with regard to issues like domestic violence or substance use or abuse, and they have to tackle subjects like mental health problems and weight gain. These rather sensitive topics are often discussed during a first antenatal visit. The reason for these questions is simply because there is evidence not only that these events happen in a woman's life, but that these can have profound effects for a woman but also for her (unborn) baby. Midwives have to ask women these sensitive questions to offer women adequate support and care. Although midwives know that asking these questions is beneficial in the long term for the health of mother and child, sometimes it feels for midwives like opening a can of worms and that they're probing in somebody's life. If the midwife has a busy antenatal clinic and little time, it can be difficult to discuss things thoroughly and to build a rapport and a relationship of trust at the same time, when the antenatal visit may be the first time the midwife and the woman meet. It can be frustrating but women's stories can sometimes be so heart breaking, that it can even have an impact on the emotions of the midwife (Mollart et al. 2009).

Reflection

Midwifery can be regarded as a maturing profession, especially for young midwives. During antenatal visits, a woman sometimes shares very private, intimate and confidential information with the midwife about what is going on in her life. These can be aspects of life that sometimes have a shocking element or are unfamiliar topics for the midwife. On the one hand, it is a privilege to be confided in by the woman – her personal thoughts, emotions and life circumstances; on the other hand, being confided in needs to be dealt with in a cautious and professional way.

A woman's story may very well include abortion, homosexual relationships, sexually transmitted diseases, drug abuse, domestic abuse or other very personal issues with a highly moral, ethically significant or social stigma. When a midwife is being confronted with difficult life issues or ethical dilemmas, at any stage of the midwife's professional development or career, it is important to reflect on his or her own ideas, values, beliefs, thoughts and feelings, and how to prevent these from influencing the midwife's care for or communication with the woman.

In difficult situations, the midwife has not only to cope with the woman's and her partner's feelings, but also with personal emotions. It is very important to be aware of personal feelings in relation to sensitive and emotionally complex situations, as well as to be able to put these aside as subordinate to the woman's opinions and emotions. It therefore needs not only professional and personal growth and development, but also a high level of self awareness and reflection from the midwife to be non-judgemental, to show that you care, sometimes to shed a tear, but also to keep a professional distance, and all at the same time. For midwifery students or young midwives it can be difficult when they seek out their friends or peers to share their experiences with or to look for comfort or a shoulder to cry on. Friends may have chosen other professions or career paths and may find it hard to understand what midwifery encompasses. Fortunately, midwives are not alone but are surrounded by other midwives and health professionals to share experiences and emotions with.

Conclusion

The word midwife means 'with women' or 'among women', sharing women's worries, their joys and their delights. To be a midwife is to engage in a close and intimate relationship, starting in pregnancy, with the effects travelling down through the centuries in the image women have of themselves, their abilities and their worth. Midwives and women are intertwined; whatever affects women affects midwives – women and midwives are interrelated and interwoven (Flint 1986 cited in Leap 2004). It is such intertwining that inspired me to become a midwife and has kept that enthusiasm going for over 20 years.

References

Buckwalter, J.G. and Simpson, S.W. (2002) 'Psychological factors in the etiology and treatment of severe nausea and vomiting in pregnancy'. *American Journal of Obstetrics and Gynecology* 186(5): S210–S214.

International Confederation of Midwives (ICM) (2005) *Definition of the Midwife*. The Hague: ICM.

Kurki, T., Hilesmaa, V., Raitasalo, R., Mattila, H. and Ylikorkala, O. (2000) 'Depression and anxiety in early pregnancy and risk for preeclampsia'. *Obstetrics & Gynecology* 95(4): 487–90.

Leap, N. (2004) 'Journey to midwifery through feminism: a personal account', in M. Stewart (ed.) *Pregnancy, Birth and Maternity Care: Feminist perspectives*. London: Elsevier Butterworth Heinemann, pp. 185–200.

Leap, N. and Homer, C. (2002) 'A strategy to teach midwifery students about woman centred care in Australia', in N. Leap, L. Barclay, P. Brodie, E. Nagy, A. Sheehan, and S. Tracy (eds) *National Review of Nursing Education: Midwifery education. Final Report, March 2002*. Sydney: Department of Education, Science and Training.

Mollart, L., Newing, C. and Foureur, M. (2009) 'Midwives' emotional wellbeing: Impact of conducting a Structured Antenatal Psychosocial Assessment (SAPSA)'. *Women and Birth* 22: 82–88.

Ross-Davie, M., Elliot, S., Sarkar, A. and Green, L. (2006) 'A public health role in perinatal mental health: Are midwives ready?' *British Journal of Midwifery* 14(6): 330–4.

Swallow, B., Lindow, S., Masson, E. and Hay, D. (2004) 'Psychological health in early pregnancy: relationship with nausea and vomiting'. *Journal of Obstetrics and Gynecology* 24(1): 28–32.

Walsh, D. and Steen, M. (2007) 'The role of the midwife: time for a review'. *Midwives* 10(7): 320–3.

Commentary

Yvonne's chapter gives us a very comprehensive picture of how the midwife in the community cares for the childbearing woman during pregnancy. The extent of this midwife's care emerges perfectly clearly. Yvonne demonstrates quite explicitly some of the variations in the experiences of women during pregnancy. What becomes disconcertingly apparent is that pregnancy may carry different meanings for the different women for whom the midwife provides care; it is not possible for the midwife to make assumptions about her women clients or to offer a routinised or 'one size fits all' approach to care. Yvonne shows us all too plainly why individualised or woman-centred care is fundamentally important in midwifery.

What also emerges from Yvonne's account is the impact of this type of work on the midwife. While Yvonne's enthusiasm for midwifery practice shines through her chapter, the difficulties which she faces in her everyday practice also manifest themselves. Practising in an area of deprivation clearly carries some challenges, in terms of relationships as well as the midwife's property. What also emerge disconcertingly clearly are some of the pressures of practising in an NHS setting; for Yvonne virtually unbearable pressure of time appears to be a fact of life. Yet it is an issue which she tells the reader she is seeking to resolve. Unfortunately, the 'sandwich at the desk' is what passes for lunch for a large proportion of NHS staff, and they may sometimes be so unlucky that they do not even get time for a sandwich. If the midwife is under such onerous pressure to complete her work, it is necessary for us to consider the effect, not only on the midwife's long-term health (Yoshida & Sandall 2013), but also on the experience of the childbearing woman and her family. I have no doubt that the midwife does everything possible to prevent the woman from realising the pressure under which she practises, but the childbearing woman may still pick up the cues.

This pressure of time may be contrasted with the service which midwives may be able to offer at other times. For example, it is only necessary to look at Chapter 10 or at what Yvonne writes in her later section on home visits.

Reference

Yoshida, Y. and Sandall, J. (2013) 'Occupational burnout and work factors in community and hospital midwives: A survey analysis'. *Midwifery* 29(8): 921–6.

3

MIDWIFERY CARE WITH THE WOMAN IN LABOUR IN AN INSTITUTION

Miranda Page

In the first edition of this book I looked at the idea of team working. This time, while touching on it, I want to take a deeper look at the issue of support. I said that I thought 'the most important quality a team needs is the ability to support each other, not only on professional matters but also emotionally with the everyday and not so everyday stresses of working in a busy unit.' So let's unpack this a little and see if support really makes a difference and if so how.

The story told in this chapter comes largely from my own experience of working in a busy urban obstetric unit, but I have also drawn on an amalgam of events and characters conjured into being through the tales of labour ward life told to me at conferences, study days and workshops, at various times in my career as a practising midwife, RCM steward and researcher. I hope, therefore, that the midwives and events I describe will ring bells and provide food for thought for practising midwives in many settings, and, for those preparing to enter the profession, an insight into hospital life through the eyes of one midwife on a typical labour ward shift.

VIGNETTE

The shift started like any other, with me in the changing rooms donning the ubiquitous hospital scrubs, which invariably were either too small or too big. Today I had a top that could've hidden an elephant and a pair of bottoms belonging to a catwalk model. Still, at least I had a pair, matching or otherwise. Ruth, my colleague, wasn't having such luck and, despite going from pleading through bribing to offering to inflict bodily harm on people in the changing room, she was forced to admit defeat. As I headed to the labour ward I saw her making for the postnatal ward to hunt down a pair of scrubs.

This particular day I was coordinating the shift. Twelve hours at the helm steering our way through hopefully calm waters with a motley crew and a precious cargo of mothers to be, new mums and babies and a few significant others thrown in for good measure.

Sue had been coordinating the night shift and, as I came through the doors, she turned her pale face towards me and smiled. Still huddled in her big woolly cardigan, she took one last sip of her now cold tea and walked with me to the duty room for report. I said a small prayer and promised that today would be different: 'Each woman that comes through that door will receive the best care. She will be valued and respected as an individual and her voice will be listened to.'

'Right, hit me with it, Sue.'

'Well,' she said, taking a deep breath and looking at the board.

'You've got three normal labourers, two inductions, one on synto, the other one's waiting for an ARM but the head's high, a forceps in theatre, a possible pre-term labourer in room 7, one in HDU with a PPH, a diabetic in room 6, two delivered in 10 and 8. But postnatal's full, so God knows where you're going to put them.' A pause, 'Oh yes, and you've got two electives due and Alice has phoned in sick again.'

'Perfect,' I sighed.

'Here's the keys.' Sue thrust a large bundle of assorted metal into my hands. 'God, I nearly forgot, you'll have to order some more morphine; we've only got ten left.' With that she picked up her bag and hurried to the door. Turning round as her hand went to the handle, she smiled again and, with thoughts of a warm bed, waved goodbye.

As she left, the motley crew arrived. Through the duty room door came the day shift – all seven of them.

'Hold on a minute,' I thought . . . 'I know Alice is off sick but that still leaves us short by two.' I cast my eyes down the staff rota.

'Where's Sam and Joan?' I demanded. 'Study day,' someone muttered from the corner.

'Who said they could go on a bloody study day?'

'You did mate,' an Antipodean voice replied. I looked up, as rushing through the door in a mismatch of pink and orange came Ruth.

'Oh bugger, yes. Still, could be worse,' I reflected. 'You've found some 'blues' then?' Martha the student midwife smirked at the back. Ruth looked on defiantly.

'Okay team,' I said, trying to put a brave face on it. 'This is going to be a bit tricky, but I'm sure we can cope with whatever's thrown at us.'

'Struth, Miranda,' Ruth exclaimed as she chewed on a breakfast roll and looked at the board. Much as I enjoyed working with this laid-back funny New Zealander, sometimes, just sometimes, I wished she would engage her brain before she opened her mouth. I shot her a 'don't frighten the juniors look' and continued to rally the troops.

'This is what we are going to do. Who's working with Martha and Heather today?' The two student midwives looked distinctly nervous at the back of the room.

'It's Jane and me.' Jane was a keen young midwife, and the 'me' was Kristy. Kristy, the labour ward Mum. Every hospital should have one. She came with the bricks and had birthed just about the whole of the county as well as five of her own. At 55 she was as wide as she was tall, a bundle of warmth and tall stories, with a large bosom who had comforted and encouraged a whole generation of midwives and doctors. And she made the meanest chocolate cake in the whole world. The two students looked relieved. In fact, we all felt better having her on shift.

'OK then, why don't you and Jane take the normal labourers and the induction in room 5?' I said brightly.

Kristy froze, narrowed her eyes and rose to her full 4 foot 11 inches and said 'Not me, duck. Me, Jane and the girls will look after . . .' and then, turning to the board, she named the women in rooms 1, 2, 3 and 4. Ruth arched an eyebrow but didn't say anything because Kristy was right. And my mantra was in tatters and we were only half an hour into the shift. Duly chastened, I resolved to do better and allocated the rest of the staff to women, not conditions.

Jo was the last to leave and she did so rather reluctantly. I knew why. I had allocated her Mrs Jones, who was in early labour and a diabetic. Now Jo was a very good midwife, but she just didn't believe in herself. She got flustered very easily and lacked confidence. A woman with complicated needs would be challenging, but I knew with support she could do it. I tried to convey this to her, but going by her mournful expression as she walked down the corridor I hadn't succeeded.

'Just come and ask me if you're worried about anything,' I called after her retreating back. Her shoulders slumped even further. Well, I had enough to worry about – trying to find postnatal beds for the women who had already had their babies and the ward round to prepare for. Was this really what I had come into midwifery to do?

'Here, doll, get this down you!' Ruth pressed a steaming mug of tea into my hand as Lucy appeared with a tray of toast.

'It could be worse,' Lucy speculated. She would say that. I don't think I'd ever seen her ruffled. Not even the day when she had three sets of twins all deciding to be born at the same time!

'How could it be worse Lucy?'

'Well,' she paused as she took a bite of buttery toast. 'You see, you're really lucky – you've got the A team working today.'

I smiled, 'But who's Mr T?'

'Mr who?' came a perky voice from behind us.

'Sweetie, you're too young to remember,' Lucy said, turning to a rather excited Jane who was practically hopping from foot to foot.

'Oh right, whatever.' Frowning, she continued, 'just popped out to let you know that room 4's starting to push.'

'You mean,' said Ruth rather ominously waving an amni-hook in Jane's direction, 'Cynthia Patterson in room 4 is feeling the urge to bear down' and, turning to us with a 'See you later girls', she made her way into her own room still, I might add, waving her amni-hook.

'Well, that's what I meant,' said the rather surprised Jane. 'Ah well,' but before Lucy could launch forth, a loud moan emanated from room 4 followed by the startled face of Martha, the student midwife.

'I think you might be wanted,' I pointed to Martha.

'Oh help,' Jane muttered and walked quickly to the door.

It shut as the dulcet tones of Cynthia Patterson rang out with 'There's no f**king way ya gonna get me to push . . . ohhhh ya bastard.'

'My, my and her a solicitor too,' commented Lucy as she went to answer the phone.

'Good morning, labour ward, Lucy Staples speaking . . . Jennifer who? . . . hold on . . .' Placing her hand over the receiver, she lent over to me and whispered, 'How's room 3 doing? It's her mum,' nodding her head at the phone.

'Room 3 . . . room 3 . . . umm . . . yes . . . Let me go and check. That's Kristy's lady, hold on.' I walked down the corridor and knocked on the door.

'Hold on . . . with you in a tick,' came the reply. I stood and thought about the million other things I should be doing rather than waiting for Kristy and tried to breathe calmly. After what seemed an age the door was flung open.

'Aye up, me duck?'

'It's her mum wants to know how she's doing,' I said by way of a reply . . .

'Doing . . . well that all depends.'

'Yes, yes I know,' I sighed, instantly regretting my turn of phrase . . . 'but what can I tell her?'

Kristy looked down at her fob watch and ruminated. 'Tell her to call back at tea time.' 'Tea time!' I exclaimed. 'But . . .' Kristy raised her left hand like a policeman stopping traffic.

'She's OP. I've put her in the bath. Teatime it will be.' And with that she turned and shut the door.

'Right you are,' I said under my breath and fast-footed it back to the phone where Lucy was looking at me expectantly.

'Tell her to call at tea time . . .'

'Hello, Mrs Adams,' said Lucy with her best telephone voice. 'The midwife looking after your daughter says to call again at tea time . . .'

'How long? . . .'

'Well, it's hard to tell . . .'

'Hopefully . . .'

'No, we can't give her something to speed it up . . .'

'Yes, I know it's been a long time . . .'

'Five days you say . . . well . . .'

'You had a drip . . . yes . . . well we try not to . . . uh uh . . .'

Lucy looked across at me and rolled her eyes.

'Just you call back at tea time and keep your fingers crossed,' she said and quickly put down the phone. It rang again straightaway; we both stared at it and then each other. Taking a deep breath I picked it up. 'Good morning, labour ward, Miranda Page speaking . . .'

'Jennifer Adams . . . and you are . . .?'

'Her mother in law . . .'

'There's no news yet . . .'

'Yes. I know it does take time doesn't it . . . How long? Well it's hard to say . . .'

'Why don't you try phoning at tea time . . .?'

'Visiting . . . no not in labour ward . . . umm. I'm sorry, you'll have to wait until she goes to the postnatal ward . . .'

'So maybe you will be able to see her tomorrow . . .'

'Between 2 and 4 and 7 and 8 in the evening . . .'

'Well, that went down like a lead balloon . . .'

'Wanted to be at the delivery, did she?' Lucy asked.

'Yes. Would you really want your mother-in-law at the birth of your baby?'

'Can't think of anything worse, darling,' Lucy pondered, but her voice trailed off as the emergency buzzer in room 7 went off.

Lucy leapt to her feet and headed to the room. Two seconds later her head reappeared and she called, 'Fast bleep the paed would you. She's pushing and there's membranes visible – won't be long.'

I picked up the receiver and started to dial just as Jo moved into my line of vision, about to ask me a question. 'Give us a sec, Jo.'

'I just wanted to ask . . .'

'Yea, yea. Hold on . . .' Answering the operator on the other end of the line, I said 'We need a paediatric registrar to labour ward, please. Thanks.' Hanging up, I said 'Sorry about that what did you . . .?' But I never got to finish the sentence because the phone rang again and it was admissions saying they had a woman coming up to labour ward pushing . . .

'Jo do us a favour; run into room 9 and see if Mary can come out and look after this woman. Tell her she's going into room . . . God, do I have a room?'

I looked about wildly in the hope that an empty room would materialise in front of me like the Tardis. It didn't, but what did was Leila, our godsend of a clinical support worker, walking beside Anne Thompson from room 8. Anne, as proud as punch carrying her new baby. Dad on the other side as white as a sheet. Trailing behind was mum. I know we are only supposed to have one partner per room but sometimes it's hard to say 'No'.

As the new family tottered down the corridor I heard Anne's mum saying to Leila, 'Well, she was a bit flat at birth. But you know the midwife just took her outside and pumped her up and now look, she's just fine; it's the happiest day of my life.' At which point she burst into tears. And off they went, barely missing the paed belting down the corridor towards them.

'What room?' he bellowed.

'7'

'Which one's that?'

I refrained from saying 'It's the one next to 6' and pointed behind him. 'That one.'

'Great.' Checking his stethoscope, which was threatening to wrap itself around his throat, he smoothed his hair down and calmly walked into the room. 'Hello there! I'm Dr Jenkins the paediatrician . . .'

Just when you think it can't get any worse, the lady from admissions appeared in a wheelchair, puffing madly . . . 'I told you we didn't have time to wait for the end of the football,' she exclaimed, whacking her husband in the chest with her handheld notes.

'Where do you want her, love?' asked the ambulance driver.

Praying that the room was clean, 'room 8,' I replied, waving vaguely in its direction. And just when you really, really don't need it – in walked the ward round.

What can you say about the ward round? It is an institution and its daily occurrence is played out in just about every obstetric labour ward in the UK. Probably in much the same way and at the same time. The entourage consisted of Dr Munroe, consultant obstetrician and soon to be Professor of Obs and Gynae, thus head honcho, surrounded by a gaggle of registrars, senior house officers (SHOs) and medical students. In all, nine more bodies cluttering up the narrow corridor that acted as the major artery running through the labour ward, which right now was in danger of bursting at the seams.

'Sister, good morning to you! And what have you got for us this morning?' He stood rubbing his hands together and rocking back and forth. Old school.

No one else called me sister. He was a big man of slightly rotund build, shall we say? And he was looking at me in anticipation. He raised an eyebrow as I was about to launch forth. I hesitated as I caught out of the corner of my eye, the fleeting figure of May Chen, our anaesthetist, bustling towards room 2. Must be for an epidural, I surmised . . . oh well . . . yes, yes, what was I saying? Dr Munroe coughed to draw my attention back to the task at hand. While I was trying to put my brain into gear, we headed to the high-dependency unit (HDU) and our lady with the PPH. 'Right, today we have Sheila Miller, a 31-year-old multigravida . . .' For the next half an hour I was preoccupied with describing the women we had in the labour ward and their many complications.

The entourage made its way around the labour ward, stopping at various rooms, where they prodded and poked, offering reassurance and dispensing advice. In between the rooms, Dr Munroe quizzed the medical students about the conditions they had just seen.

When we arrived at Jo's room, I was relieved to see her looking a little less frazzled. But I was also struck with guilt as I remembered she had been desperate to ask me something. I looked at her, trying to convey an apology. 'Did you manage to get some help?' I mouthed, as Dr Munroe, the registrars, SHOs and medical students squeezed into the room. Was it really possible to get 13 people into one tiny labour room, and that's including the poor woman and her partner? Oh, and Ruth.

Ruth was bending over one of the many pumps attached to Cath Wright, our 'diabetic'. 'That should do you now,' she said, tapping on the screen at the front of the contraption.

'Thanks so much.' Jo heaved a sigh of relief.

'No worries. Onwards and upwards, and while you're here,' Ruth said, turning her attention to 'the posse', as she liked to call the ward round. 'You don't need to come to my room. We're doing absolutely fine. I'll give you a shout if we need you . . . OK mate?' she ended, directing her gaze at the soon-to-be Prof.

'Absolutely . . . right sister . . . of course.'

Ruth exited the room, but I distinctly heard her muttering, 'Do I look like a bleeding nun?'

I left the group with Jo giving an update on Cath Wright's progress and popped my head out into the corridor. You never know what might happen when your back's turned. All seemed remarkably quiet. The faint whiff of toast lingered in the air, a sign that a baby had just arrived. It mingled with the smell of disinfectant and the distinct aroma of boiled cabbage. You can't beat that hospital smell.

The sun must have been shining, as the afterglow of light filtered through the glass panel of the sluice door – the only light that reached the labour ward corridor. Footsteps echoed around the corner and the slow grating metal on metal of an erratic trolley added to the eerie air of calm.

A small 'ping ping bong' sound caught my attention. I saw the door of room 7 open and, coming out, pushed by the paed, an incubator with our latest arrival going to the neonatal unit around the corner. It was closely followed by dad clutching a mobile and a sheet of paper with a list of names to phone. He looked rather shaken but smiled at me as he passed.

'Four pounds,' he said in amazement. 'Thanks so much.'

The day progressed in much the same way. Jo cheered up and she looked positively happy when I saw her ensconced in the treatment room with our new registrar, calculating Cath's insulin regime. Nice to see doctors and midwives working so well together, I thought in passing.

By teatime, Lucy and I were back at the desk surveying the damage. We had just about cleared the board by 5 p.m., but it was beginning, as always, to fill up again. Jane had had three deliveries and was sitting resting her feet, while Martha, her student, was eyeing up the box of chocolates that lay unopened on the desk.

'Go on, open them! You know you want to,' Jane said as the phone rang. Lucy stretched a rather weary arm out.

'Labour ward. Lucy Staples speaking. How can I help?'

She looked up at me and nodded towards Kristy's room. 'Any news yet?'

'I'll just go and check.' Finding it rather difficult to rouse myself, I moved from my chair and wandered down the corridor. Heather answered the door. Behind her shoulder I could see the huddled shapes of Sarah Adams, still in the pool, her baby snuggled into her chest and dad kneeling behind with his arms around them both.

They were cocooned in a velvety light washed over by soft music. I could just make out Kristy sitting in a rocking chair – peacefully filling in her notes. She looked up and smiled. Giving Heather the thumbs up, I gently closed the door. Coming back to the desk, I said to Lucy 'Tell her that someone will be phoning very shortly.'

So that was that really. A typical day for us, but one of the most memorable and special for the women we were caring for. Just before 8 p.m. the door opened and Sue walked in.

'All right girls,' she said. I picked up the keys to make my way to the duty room after her. 'Oh God,' I yelped, making everyone jump.

'The morphine. I've forgot to order the ruddy morphine . . .'

It's Okay doll. I did it this afternoon.'

'Ruth, I could kiss you.'

'Steady on mate.'

Supporting the team

Turning to the midwifery literature on 'peer support' runs us into a dead end. Going to the usual suspects in terms of search engines, 'Cumulative Index of Nursing and Allied Health Literature' (CINAHL), Medline, etc., using 'support' and 'midwife' or 'support and midwifery' brings up articles that invariably focus on the support midwives give to women and their families, and little on how we support each other. When support is raised in this context articles focus on the role of supervision, which according to Mander (2001) is often anything but supportive. Broadening out and looking at nursing research on support and in the wider disciplines of Management and Organisational Behaviour we find an extensive body of work examining the role of support on job satisfaction and workplace stress, so this might be a good place to start.

In the management literature support is often examined from three viewpoints: perceived organisational support (POS) (Aselage and Eisenberger 2003), perceived supervisory support (PSS) and perceived co-worker support (PCS) (Ng and Sorensen 2008). Their findings show that perceived support at each level has a strong impact on workers' sense of well-being and job satisfaction (Van Emmerik *et al.* 2007; Ng and Sorensen 2008).

Relating these findings to the vignette, we can see how different types of stress pervade the midwives' day and how the individual responses to these stressors impact on the effectiveness of the team and the care they are able to give to women and their families.

I turn first to perceived organisational support, which has been defined as the employee's beliefs about how much the organisation cares and values them. In a midwifery context there are many examples of where there appears to be a dissonance between the individual's practice beliefs and values and that of the organisation in which they work (Green 2005; Page and Mander 2014). In these situations there is increased stress as the individual struggles to adapt her practice to conform to the norms of the organisation. This conflict will often lead to the individual feeling undervalued by the organisation. In a similar vein, Babin and Boles (1996) examine the impact of stress on the individual when there is a gap between organisational expectations of their role and the customers' expectations; in midwifery read the women's needs and expectations. However, what the midwifery literature does not offer is an explanation of how this stress can be reduced. We have to turn to nursing and management literature to find that managing these pressures requires developing a range of coping mechanisms, one of which is having recourse to social support.

Defining social support is a little ambiguous in the literature but it would seem that social support in the workplace has attributes of shared experience, sympathy and compassion (Heaney *et al.* 1995). It also seems to be connected to trusting, non-judgemental and non-blaming attitudes (Mackin and Sinclair 1998).

Looking at the role of supervisory and co-worker support we find many similarities. Positive support from supervisors is conceptualised as the degree to which employees feel supervisors provide instrumental (work-related information and feedback) and emotional assistance (Ng and Sorensen 2008). Often it is assumed to be of equal value to the support offered by co-workers, where emotional support of shared experiences and compassion is thought to have a buffering effect on work stress (Mackin and Sinclair 1998). However, Ng and Sorensen (2008) argue that positive support from supervisors should be of higher value since it should be part of their role and, therefore, they should be better skilled at delivering support, and more constant in that delivery. Again turning to the midwifery literature, there are many examples of poor supervisory interactions (Kirkham 1999; Leap 1997; Ball *et al.* 2002). Therefore in the absence of supervisory support, employees turn to their colleagues for many of the same qualities of social support denied them from higher up the ladder.

Studies have also found that there is an inverse relationship between stress and quality of care (Aiken *et al.* 2001), so that as levels of stress increase the ability to deliver quality care goes down. Reducing stress therefore becomes vital, not just for the individual and organisation, since working with high levels of stress leads to reduced job satisfaction and well-being, as well as higher staff turnover (Abualrub *et al.* 2009; Rodwell *et al.* 2009), but of equal importance, it makes it more difficult to care, which in a caring profession is rather crucial.

Having a positive support mechanism enables people to better manage their stress, giving them value in their role and lightening the physical and intellectual demands of the job. Giving and receiving compassion between co-workers and supervisors in the work setting increases well-being and caring capabilities (Ashker *et al.* 2012). Given that midwifery is an emotionally 'bounded' profession (Hunter 2005), it is not unreasonable to translate these findings and set them within the context of childbirth (Leinweber and Rowe 2010).

It is with this in mind that I hope I have shown, through the example of an eventful shift, that the care and compassion shown by and to co-workers, which is not always easy in a busy unit, is not some soft add-on, some 'touchy feely' item on a wish list, but a crucial part of our ability to care for women. So the laughter, banter and relationships formed in this story play a vital part in who we are as midwives. This is because it enables us to better care for ourselves, each other and, most importantly, women, their babies and their families.

References

Abualrub, R.F., Omari, F.H., and Abu Al Rub, A.F. (2009) 'The moderating effect of social support on the stress-satisfaction relationship among Jordanian hospital nurses'. *Journal of Nursing Management* 17: 870–8.

Aiken, L.H., Clarke, S.P., Sloane, D.M., Sochalski, J.A., Busse, R., Clarke, H., *et al.* (2001) 'Nurse's reports on hospital care in five countries'. *Health Affairs* 20: 185–96.

Aselage, J. and Eisenberger, R. (2003) 'Perceived organizational support and psychological contracts: A theoretical integration'. *Journal of Organizational Behavior* 24: 491–501.

Ashker, V.E., Penprase, B. and Salman, A. (2012) 'Work-related emotional stressors and coping strategies that affect the well-being of nurses working in hemodialysis units'. *Nephrology Nursing Journal* 39(3): 231–7.

Babin, B.J. and Boles, J.S. (1996) 'The effects of perceived co-worker involvement and supervisor support on service provider role stress, performance and job satisfaction'. *Journal of Retailing* 72: 57–75.

Ball, L., Curtis P. and Kirkham, M. (2002) 'Why do midwives leave?' Women's Informed Childbearing and Health Research Group, University of Sheffield.

Green, B. (2005) 'Midwives' coping methods for managing birth uncertainties'. *British Journal of Midwifery* 13(5): 293–8.

Heaney, C.A., Price, R.H. and Rafferty, J. (1995) 'Increasing coping resources at work: A field experiment to increase social support, improve work team functioning, and enhance employee mental health'. *Journal of Organizational Behaviour* 16: 335–52.

Hunter, B. (2005) 'Emotion work and boundary maintenance in hospital based midwifery'. *Midwifery* 21: 253–66.

Kirkham, M. (1999) 'The culture of midwifery in the National Health Service in England'. *Journal of Advanced Nursing* 30(3): 732–9.

Leap, N. (1997) 'Birthwrite. Making sense of "horizontal violence" in midwifery'. *British Journal of Midwifery* 5(11): 689.

Leinweber, J. and Rowe, H.J. (2010) The costs of "being with the woman": secondary traumatic stress in midwifery'. *Midwifery* 26: 76–87.

Mackin, P. and Sinclair, M. (1998) 'Labour ward midwives perceptions of stress'. *Journal of Advanced Nursing* 27(5): 986–91.

Mander, R. (2001) *Supportive Care and Midwifery*. Oxford: Blackwell Science.

Ng, T.W.H. and Sorensen, K.L. (2008) 'Towards a further understanding of the relationships between perceptions of support and work attitudes: A meta-analysis'. *Group and Organization Management* 33: 243, originally published online 1 February 2008. doi: 1177/1059601107313307, accessed 15 February 2013.

Page, M. and Mander, R. (2014) 'Intrapartum uncertainty: A feature of normal birth, as experienced by midwives in Scotland'. *Midwifery* 30(1): 28–35.

Rodwell, J., Noblet, A., Demir, D. and Steane, P. (2009) 'Supervisors are central to work characteristics affecting nurse outcomes'. *Journal of Nursing Scholarship* 41(3): 310–19.

Van Emmerik, I.J.H., Euwema, M.C. and Bakker, A.B. (2007) 'Threats of workplace violence and the buffering effect of social support'. *Group and Organization Management* 32: 152–75.

Commentary

Miranda's chapter begins in an almost humorous fashion but as the complexities of everyday work in a labour ward catering for women in normal labour to those with multifaceted problems unfold it turns into a dramatic theatre rivalling the most fast-moving films. While the meaning of midwife is generally understood as being 'with woman', this snapshot of one shift shows how this must be interpreted much more widely. This midwife is not just required to be with a woman but to be with several through her effective coordination of the clinical area. Have her midwifery skills in being with woman prepared her for the management role she must undertake or have these come from some further education? Is this role of coordinator a natural progression from supporting one woman to supporting several labouring women as well as more junior midwives and students hoping to become midwives?

Mackin and Sinclair (1999) and Kirkham (2011) highlighted similar issues but these appear not to have been researched further. The multifaceted issue remains somewhat mysterious and of course is variable from day to day. While it would have been much less dramatic to have highlighted a quieter day in the same labour ward, the outcomes for both the women and the midwives involved may have been much more palpable. However, in no less a way are these also so dependent on the expertise and competence of the senior midwife coordinating the shift.

References

Kirkham, M. (2011) 'The role of the midwife with the woman in labour: to be with, to monitor or to wait on the landing?' *MIDIRS Midwifery Digest* 21(4): 469–70.

Mackin, P. and Sinclair, M. (1999) 'Midwives' experience of stress on the labour ward'. *British Journal of Midwifery* 7(5): 323 6.

4

MIDWIFERY CARE OF THE MOTHER AND BABY AT HOME

Allison Ewing

VIGNETTE

It is now 30 years since I embarked on my journey to be a midwife. As a student nurse in 1984, I saw that first-time mothers were kept in hospital for the full statutory 10 days! This seems astonishing now, but was necessary as there were not enough midwives to provide community postnatal care. The district nurses were both qualified nurses as well as midwives, commanding a higher salary than some of their hospital counterparts, and didn't have enough time to provide both nursing and midwifery care. Mothers in subsequent pregnancies were 'allowed' out after four days. Fortunately, this did appear to give the women a good grounding in breastfeeding and basic baby care before they went home. As is pointed out later in the chapter, the UK was almost unique in providing midwifery care at home when women were discharged from hospital.

In 2009, I contributed to the first edition of this book and now have been asked to revise this chapter for the second edition. My first thought when I was asked was that the chapter would be very short and should be retitled 'Postnatal Midwifery Care: Rest In Peace'. In 2009, I detailed how we would need to 'fight for the protection of one of the jewels of the midwifery service in the UK' as Evans had pleaded in 2001. In too many places in the UK, the fight has been lost, in the name of shrinking resources and 'austerity Britain'. This is also the case in other countries in Europe where insurance companies are reducing the number of funded visits by midwives to women during the postnatal period.

In 2009 I illustrated the chapter with vignettes of actual practice highlighting the value of skilful, knowledgeable continuity of midwifery care, with one detailing the importance in detecting sepsis. This year I will be writing of another instance when midwifery vigilance succeeded in detecting a maternal complication which may have led to a more severe consequence.

In 2011, the Centre for Maternal and Child Enquiries (CMACE) reported that the leading cause of maternal death in the UK for the 3 years from 2006 to 2008 was genital tract sepsis. This is the first time since 1952 that the leading cause of death has been from this cause.

I make no apologies that I will, as in the last edition, go back to basics to highlight why and how traditional British midwifery care encompassed care of the mother and baby in the home and why I still believe it is an essential part of midwifery care. Potential midwives reading this may wonder why I am delving into the historic past, but with the programme and book of *Call The Midwife* (Worth 2007, BBC 2012) causing an increase in applicants for midwifery courses, I believe you should know the history of our profession.

Historical basis of community based postnatal care

What is, or was postnatal care? When midwifery care was regulated at the beginning of the twentieth century, one of the main causes of mortality and morbidity of women and babies was either maternal or neonatal sepsis. Until 1986 there was a statutory requirement in the Midwives' Rules for midwives to visit the woman daily until 10 days, with a recommendation that the woman have two visits a day in the first few days if she had given birth at home (Sweet 1983; Garcia *et al.* 1994). In the tenth edition of *Mayes' Midwifery* (Sweet 1983), the chapter on postnatal complications is mostly concerned with the detection, by the midwife, of postnatal infections in the mother and in the baby.

The midwife would therefore be taking the pulse and temperature of the postnatal woman regularly to assess if there was a developing fever. She would be assessing the breasts and nipples for any sign of trauma from breastfeeding as this could lead to mastitis and breast abscess. She would enquire about vaginal discharge (lochia) for colour, odour and amount. In 'top to toe' examination she would then be palpating the uterus to detect if it was involuting (returning to its normal size and location in the pelvic cavity) and whether it was tender to touch. Next might be a question about passing urine and opening bowels. Urinary tract infection might be a risk as there is dilatation of the ureter in pregnancy and the woman may have difficulty in fully emptying her bladder. This can result in some urine remaining in the urinary tract allowing bacteria to grow. The woman might also be reluctant to pass urine if she has grazes or other trauma to the genital area. Her perineum would be inspected if she had sustained damage to it to assess healing. Finally she would be asked about her legs, as there would be a perceived risk of thromboembolism. This is because after the birth, the blood becomes more viscous again as the excess fluid that has been in the cardiovascular system in pregnancy is excreted soon after the baby is born. Women with a previous history of varicose veins would be at more risk. Thromboembolism was also probably more prevalent as a result of the advice for the woman to be nursed in bed.

The midwife would then turn her attention to the baby. Sleeping, feeding and excreting habits would be enquired about. She might then, at least twice in the period of her visits, perform a 'top to toe' examination to assess colour of the baby (looking for jaundice) and tone. She would be looking at the eyes, mouth, skin and umbilicus for signs of infection as in the mother. For the midwife then, 'cleanliness was next to Godliness' and great care was to be taken to prevent infection with thorough hand washing the most important (Sweet 1983).

If this was a first-time mother, the midwife might then demonstrate how to 'top and tail' the baby, bath the baby, give breastfeeding support or show how to make up a bottle feed safely. This would give the new mother a good grounding in basic care of the newborn. One advantage that the midwife and mother had was that they would likely know each other, as there was a good chance that the midwife would have provided the antenatal care as well as being present at the birth.

Very little is written in Sweet (1983) about the emotional and mental wellbeing of the mother, with only two pages devoted to 'Psychiatric Disorders'. On page 413 can be found the following:

> A calm and placid woman, happily married and secure, may weather the emotional storms of pregnancy, labour and the puerperium without more than an occasional attack of 'blues'. One who is temperamentally more anxious and nervous may find the same degree of emotional strain intolerable. For the woman with a history of mental instability the stress of pregnancy and labour may initiate a recurrence of mental illness.

This is in marked contrast to, 20 years later, the detailed chapter in the fourteenth edition of the Myles *Textbook for Midwives* (Fraser and Cooper 2003) which addresses this issue and which is discussed in more detail in Chapter 5 of this book.

In the mid part of the twentieth century the community midwife was seen as a valued and integral part of the community. Worth (2007) and Joyce (2008) have both written vivid and moving memoirs of midwifery care in the 50s and 60s. It is not altogether a rosy picture and there was a great deal of poverty and deprivation in the areas in which they worked; the work depicted was demanding and hard. The community midwife in those times was also, usually, a midwifery sister and would have a higher salary than most of her hospital counterparts to reflect the greater clinical responsibility in attending 'home confinements'.

After the Peel Report in 1970 and the recommendation that all births should be in hospital, the role of the community midwife was vastly reduced to consist mostly of staffing antenatal clinics and performing postnatal visits. The deskilling of midwives who could attend home births continued. At this time it would be highly unlikely that a midwife would be attending a woman she knew in labour although there might be good continuity of care and carer in the ante- and postnatal period.

In the late 80s and early 90s there was a resurgence in midwives trying to reclaim midwifery in the community with initiatives such as the Know Your Midwife scheme founded by Caroline Flint and the One To One scheme instigated by Lesley Page, now president of The Royal College of Midwives. Both of these projects were attempting to provide more continuity of care and carer in the whole of the pregnancy, labour and postnatal period (Page 2003).

With the Flint scheme, the aim was that the woman would have met the midwife attending her in labour at least once in the antenatal period. I was fortunate to work in the first NHS roll-out of this scheme in the early 90s being in a team of six midwives who were all earning the same salary. It was an exciting time to be working and was manageable when there was a realistic caseload for the team and the team was of a small enough size for effective communication and cooperation. There was great job satisfaction as a midwife, but a mother might have felt that there was less continuity of carer in the postnatal period as all members of the team took it in turns to staff the antenatal clinics, be on call for labour and perform the postnatal visits. The team ran coffee mornings for groups of women due in the same month so that they could meet each other and get to know the whole team.

The Page One to One scheme has now become known as Caseload Midwifery and for many midwives and mothers this can provide the ideal way to work and be cared for. For this to work, though, there has to be a realistic caseload. This will be discussed more in the next section.

That was then, this is now

So how have things changed now? What are the challenges facing the average community midwife today?

I would say that one of the biggest challenges to the modern community midwife now is that there are not enough of them to go round. There is a recognised shortage of midwives in many parts of the UK. Numbers are debated by government and the Royal College of Midwives (RCM) but the reality is that there are fewer whole time equivalent (WTE) midwives than there were 20 years ago. There was a drop of 5,000 in the number of practising midwives between 1992 and 2003 (NMC 2004). The introduction of more family-friendly employment policies and parity of pay and conditions between part-time and full-time workers has encouraged more midwives, especially those with young families, to work part time. Also, some midwives without children might simply choose to work part time to relieve stress at work. So, while numbers of midwives might look the same on paper, there are still too few WTE.

As maternity services are centralised, the concentration of births in the large obstetric units has also meant that when there is a shortage of midwives, the remaining ones will need to be concentrated in the high-risk and potentially litigious area of intrapartum care. So where does that leave community postnatal care if most of the midwives are in the hospital?

After the 10-day statutory requirement was removed in the 80s, selective visiting slowly became the norm. Part of the rationale for the removal of the statutory requirement was that in some cases, midwives were visiting some women who were not at home and thus not seen to be in need of midwifery services. This was obviously a waste of the midwives' time and the NHS's money. The introduction of the selective visiting was supposed to be in partnership and agreement with the needs of the mother and was generally welcomed by midwives.

In many cases it started with the woman being visited daily for approximately the first 4 days and then on alternative days till day 10 when care would be handed over to the health visitor. The Midwives' Rules still maintained that a midwife could visit up till 28 days, but the midwife would have to demonstrate a good reason why a woman might still be 'on the books' after 10 days. Her time management skills might be called into question if she could not manage to see 12 postnatal women and run a 2-hour antenatal clinic in an 8-hour day.

It is deeply depressing to report that this slippery slope to the erosion of midwifery postnatal care has taken an even steeper incline. In many places in England where the midwifery shortage has bitten deep, many women are only getting one or two visits in the 10-day period. These visits are functional to weigh the baby and to take the heel prick test, which tests for several different metabolic disorders, which, if caught early, can be treated. This happens despite the fact that hospitals with fewer beds than 20 years ago are having to discharge women as quickly as possible back into the community. In this time it was expected that, between visits, the woman would be able to recognise if there were any problems with herself or her baby and be able to contact a midwife if necessary.

An example from the field shows some of the potential dangers. All names used are pseudonyms.

Sheila, an independent midwife, has attended the successful home birth of Jane. This is Jane's second birth with Sheila. Sheila has visited on days 1, 2, 3 and 5 postpartum. On day 5 she weighs the baby and performs the heel prick test. She has practised selective visiting but this woman is an experienced mother and the decision to miss some days has been a joint one. Now, in the current format of standard postnatal care in some areas, this might be when the visits by the midwife stop, but Sheila has the 'luxury' of being able to give more time and individualised care to Jane and her baby and arranges to come back on day 7. The baby has been slightly jaundiced but not enough to interfere with breastfeeding or excretion. When the midwife returns on day 7, Jane reports that the baby has been more sleepy and reluctant to feed. The jaundice is not any worse, in fact, if anything it looks better. The midwife cannot put her finger on what is wrong with the baby. The baby's temperature is 37.5, heart beat is 140 and respirations are 40. The woman's other child has a respiratory virus and has not gone to nursery. The midwife inspects the umbilicus: clean and healing with no sign of inflammation. She pulls down the nappy and there she finds a small 50p sized lesion/blister just on the right groin looking red and inflamed, with some pus in the centre. The mother had not noticed it being there when she had changed the nappy a couple of hours earlier. The midwife recommends that the baby be seen at the local children's hospital. Jane waits for her husband to come home, goes to the hospital, the baby is admitted and has intravenous antibiotics for four days for scalded skin syndrome caused by staphylococcus aureus, which was beginning to become a systemic infection.

There are two questions I would like to ask:

1   What might have happened had that woman been having a standard visiting pattern?
2   She was an experienced mother and might have been expected to notice something like that. Why didn't she?

The baby was discharged on oral antibiotics after 4 days, had continued to breastfeed in hospital and luckily did not get thrush as a result of taking the antibiotics. Sheila was able to continue to give care in tandem with the health visitor until she was satisfied that the baby was on the mend. Sheila did not fully discharge this mother and her baby from her care till day 32. He continues to thrive. It would seem that the role of the midwife in detecting postnatal infections might still be needed.

Unfortunately, some cases of postnatal infection are being missed or dismissed (BBC 2008). A midwife was struck off the NMC register in December 2008 for failing to spot that a woman was developing a septicaemia. The woman subsequently died. On reading the report and related articles, it transpires that the woman had been seen by two other midwives and a GP before being visited by the midwife in question. The midwife had been placed on 'conditions of practice' following the death of the mother, but had subsequently made more mistakes. The midwife's GP had made a statement that she had been suffering from post-traumatic stress disorder and depression during the period since the death.

More questions:

1   Would continuity of carer have had any effect on the outcome?
2   The midwife had also been a community midwife for many years. Without wanting to excuse her actions in any way, what changes in her working pattern may she have experienced in her working life? How much time were the midwives able to spend on the visits?

It is now time, I think, to return to the comment I made at the beginning of the chapter about the fact that the most common cause of maternal death between 2006 and 2008 was sepsis, and use another example from the field.

Would lack of continuity have had a different outcome?

VIGNETTE

Sheila has been caring for Chloe and her husband Simon. They booked her fairly late in the pregnancy but Chloe has had comprehensive antenatal care and has had every available screening test. Chloe has been anxious and has asked her GP to refer her to Perinatal Mental Health Services. This he does, but the psychiatrist determines that there is no sign of pathological mental illness and tells her to carry on but if any further concerns, to come back.

Meanwhile, the pregnancy continues and Chloe proceeds to have an uncomplicated homebirth with Sheila and her colleague. It is noted at the birth, however, that there were some abnormalities in the placenta. There had been absolutely no signs of fetal distress.

Sheila arranges to come back 12 hours after the birth and there are no problems found at this visit. She arranges to come back next day, and this time, 33 hours after the birth, the baby is very jaundiced and has not been feeding very well. After a difficult time trying to contact a relevant senior midwife or supervisor of midwives, she arranges for the baby to be reviewed at the local hospital. The upshot of this is that the baby is admitted to the special care baby unit by the duty registrar. The next day, the consultant paediatrician picks up a heart murmur which had been missed at admission and the baby is referred to the local children's hospital where a major heart defect is diagnosed. The parents are understandably distraught as during pregnancy they had had a detailed anomaly ultrasound which had not picked up this abnormality.

As the baby is now being cared for in the appropriate place, it is now Sheila's job to care for and support Chloe and Simon. Understandably the parents are spending most of their time at the hospital. As Sheila is an independent midwife, she is unable to provide clinical care in the hospital setting but hopes that Chloe will be examined by the hospital staff (as she had been booked at the hospital before engaging Sheila) but later finds out that this has not happened. When the couple finally get home for an evening, Sheila is able to go and make her examination on day 3. All is physically well and Chloe remains physically well until day 6 when she calls Sheila to say that she is feeling unwell, has a stiff neck, feels shivery and has diarrhoea. When Sheila gets there, she finds that Chloe is apyrexial, but has a uterus which is tender on palpation and she detects a slight odour. At the birth, Sheila had noted that the membranes had been ragged and had been vigilant for signs of infection. She takes a swab from the vagina and arranges for Chloe to get antibiotics from the GP. The uterus remains tender for a few days but then starts to involute normally again. Like the previous case from the field, Sheila was also able to continue to care for the mother and the baby (when discharged from hospital) until 31 days postnatal. She was able to monitor Chloe's emotional well-being and communicate with GP, HV and psychiatrist when she discharged them.

A few weeks later, Sheila learns that a woman in the same city developed a puerperal sepsis and died around about the same time that Sheila had been caring for Chloe.

In the CMACE (2011) report on page 87 there is a graph showing the upward trend in genital tract sepsis since 1985. The incidence has doubled. Although it might just be a coincidence, I would remind you that it was in 1986 that the statutory requirement for postnatal visits for 10 days was abolished.

So what does CMACE recommend to stem this rise?

I attended one of the conferences for the publication of the report and was deeply disappointed to hear a very senior midwife recommend that all the women should be given a thermometer! I would remind you that Sheila's client was not pyrexial and sometimes, usually well women may be severely ill before they succumb to the infection and may demonstrate idiosyncratic symptoms.

CMACE also recommend the use of a MEWS (Maternal Early Warning) chart. Now I would suggest that this is because the majority of the postnatal care, if any, might be fragmented and undertaken by untrained and unregulated health care support workers who might be able to take basic clinical observations, but might lack the background knowledge and experience to interpret them.

Half of the deaths were from Group A Beta Haemolytic Streptococcus and the report was at pains to state that this is 'typically community based' and that 'historically it is the classic organism associated with puerperal sepsis and was a major cause of maternal mortality before antiseptic practice was introduced and antibiotics became available.' (CMACE 2011 p. 88). I would submit that if this organism is 'community based' then MORE community staff should be made available.

The report advocates emphasising the teaching, in the antenatal period, of the importance of good personal hygiene and hand washing. When is this going to happen if antenatal education is reduced? When is teaching going to happen in the postnatal ward when women and their babies are discharged soon after delivery and there are no community staff to teach them? Give them a leaflet? Well, that is what they do get and I have been told by several women that many of these and similar leaflets are just put in the bin.

In England, at present, there are still some bastions of the model of caseload midwifery care, but they are coming under threat. Shortly after the publication of the first edition of this book, the long-established, well-respected and lauded Albany Team Midwives who were contracted into King's College Hospital Trust in London, were closed down on dubious grounds. The Albany midwives were unique in that, as they were contracted in, they had more autonomy and freedom to practice than the other directly employed group practices at King's.

However, it would appear that even these other successful caseload practices may be under threat as their 'outcomes' and 'working patterns' are now being scrutinised after the appointment of a new director of midwifery (private anonymous correspondence, May 2013). These practices would be seen as quite anomalous as the individuals employed in them still have the freedom to see their clients with their discretion and up to 28 days postnatal instead of the one or two postnatal visits which have become the norm in other areas.

The future?

Four years ago I was pessimistic about the future of community midwifery postnatal care and that has not changed. The language used in the first section of this chapter was deliberately archaic and formal to reflect the teaching and expectations of the time. The twenty-first century textbook now talks about the midwife helping in the transition and adaptation to parenthood and working in partnership with the woman (Marchant 2003). A lot more emphasis is now placed on the emotional and mental well-being of the mother, as well it should (Raynor and Oates 2003).

There is criticism that the 'top to toe' examination may not give the woman space to articulate her real concerns, but this back-to-basics approach may be desperately needed to help stem the rise in deaths. However, in order for the woman to be able to articulate her feelings, the time taken for the examination may help her to feel comfortable with the midwife to be able to express herself.

Towards the end of my time as a community midwife in the NHS, the time constraints were becoming tighter and I was spending less time on postnatal visits. It was frustrating to know that if I wanted to get round all my visits I would not want to find any 'problems' which would need action or take time. I did not always have the time to spend with a woman to assist in breastfeeding or to notice any clues that she might want to talk about anything.

I had been a midwife for six years before I became a mother and until then I had not truly appreciated the value of having community postnatal care. I was also doubly lucky that I had been cared for by two of my friends and colleagues and had not truly appreciated the value of continuity of care and carer until that time. I am absolutely sure that my birth and my adaptation to motherhood would have been quite different had I experienced fragmented care. As an aside, in a nearby hospital, midwives are now banned from caring for colleagues, friends or relatives.

In the first edition I talked about the increased stress in our profession and the feeling of being undervalued and I'm afraid, this has got much, much worse. There has been a change of government and a major change in the provision of health care in England and it is too early to predict what will happen to English maternity services when the profitable services have been taken over by private companies. At the conference we were told that CMACE was being disbanded and it is unclear what has succeeded this. Will the new private companies be willing to continue to contribute to these confidential enquiries? They may not be subject to freedom of information requests.

Maybe my comments at the end of this chapter may appear to have gone off topic, but I would urge any of you reading this and thinking of becoming a midwife to really think about the politics and the psychology of midwifery care as well as the very important physiology. What is midwifery to you? To me, it was, and still is, the care of the woman and the baby through the whole of the pregnancy, birth and postnatal period. Unfortunately, in Britain, we are now losing this, as most clinical midwives are confined to the busy delivery wards. Perhaps, if you really want to be 'with woman', you might need to be a doula or a maternity care assistant.

References

BBC News Channel (2008) 'Midwife struck off after death'. http://news.bbc.co.uk/1/hi/wales/7775755.stm. Accessed 12 January 2009.

BBC Productions (2012) *Call the Midwife*.

Centre for Maternal and Child Enquiries (CMACE) (2011) *Saving Mothers' Lives: Reviewing Maternal Deaths to Make Motherhood Safer: 2006–08*. The Eighth Report on the Confidential Enquiries into Maternal Deaths in the United Kingdom. *BJOG* 118 (Suppl. 1): 1–203.

Evans, J. (2001) 'Woman-centred postnatal care: the personal view of an independent midwife'. *MIDIRS Midwifery Digest* 1: S7–S8.

Fraser, D.M. and Cooper M.A. (eds) (2003) *Myles Textbook for Midwives*, 14th edition. Edinburgh: Churchill Livingstone.

Garcia, J., Renfrew, M. and Marchant, S. (1994) 'Postnatal home visiting by midwives'. *Midwifery* 10(1): 40–43.

Joyce, H. (2008) *The Green Lady. Memoirs of a Glasgow Midwife*. Circle 49 Publishing Association, Canada.

Marchant, S. (2003) 'The puerperium', in D.M. Fraser and M.A. Cooper (eds), *Myles Textbook for Midwives*, 14th edition. Edinburgh: Churchill Livingstone.

Nursing and Midwifery Council (NMC) (2004) *Statistical Analysis of the Register*. http://www.nmc-uk.org/Documents/Statistical%20analysis%20of%20the%20register/NMC%20Statistical%20analysis%20of%20the%20register%202002%202003.pdf

Page, L. (2003) 'Woman-centred, midwife-friendly care: principles, patterns and culture of practice', in D.M. Fraser and M.A. Cooper (eds), *Myles Textbook for Midwives*, 14th edition. Edinburgh: Churchill Livingstone.

Raynor, M.D. and Oates, M.R. (2003) 'The psychology and psychopathology of pregnancy and childbirth', in D.M. Fraser and M.A. Cooper (eds), *Myles Textbook for Midwives*, 14th edition. Edinburgh: Churchill Livingstone.

Sweet, B.R. (1983) *Mayes' Midwifery. A Textbook for Midwives*, 10th edition. London: Baillere Tindall.

Worth, J. (2007) *Call The Midwife. A true story of the East End in the 1950s*. London: Weidenfeld & Nicolson.

Commentary

It comes as no surprise that Allison's take on community midwifery care represents a highly politicised picture of the community midwife's practice. Her focus on the less than glamorous but disconcertingly frequent infectious conditions presents a clarion call to all who provide care to the woman and her baby. Although her 'Back to Basics' message may have suffered from some over-exposure among hypocritical politicians, it should still underpin much midwifery practice.

Allison correctly calls our attention to the place of the midwife in a national system of health care. While the concept of the National Health Service when legislation was passed in 1946 provided a beacon of how health care should be provided, attitudes have changed, resulting in expectations of a first-class service at bargain basement prices. The upshot is that staff, such as the community midwife, seek to provide that service at a cost to their own health, as mentioned by Yvonne in Chapter 2.

The expectation that the new mother should be alert to inform the midwife of problems developing, both in her baby's and her own body, is less than realistic. Even the experienced mother is likely to be challenged at having to care for her new baby 24/7, as well as what she probably feels are her obligations to the other family members. The extent and depth of the problem of tiredness after the birth (Cooklin *et al.* 2012) are such that the mother cannot be expected to anticipate them. It is for the community midwife, though, to help the woman to identify both help and coping strategies at this supremely challenging time.

It is such apparently basic, but actually insoluble, problems that are faced by the midwife. The media and the chattering classes may admire the costly hi-tech medical interventions which may assist a small number of women and their babies. The reality of seeking to support the new mother through the rigours of the early days and weeks is considerably less sophisticated and falls to the midwife.

Reference

Cooklin, A.R., Giallo, R. and Rose, N. (2012) 'Parental fatigue and parenting practices during early childhood: an Australian community survey'. *Child: Care, Health and Development* 38(5): 654–64.

PART 2

The midwife and the wider environment

5

MIDWIVES AND PERINATAL MENTAL HEALTH

Eleanor Forrest

VIGNETTE

Emma's friend, Ros, has noticed that, since becoming pregnant, Emma has been very nervous and pre-occupied. Emma is now 12 weeks pregnant. Ros talks with Emma, who confides that she is really worried about the baby. This is because Emma had a lot of alcohol to drink around the time she fell pregnant. Now Emma can't sleep properly, has difficulty concentrating and feels nervous all the time.

Although the exact reasons are not entirely clear, stress and anxiety in pregnancy can have adverse effects. These adverse effects include premature labour, separation of the placenta, low infant birth weight and the baby being born in a poor condition. Pregnant women such as Emma who experience similar anxieties and concerns and mild to moderate levels of anxiety are common and are linked with physical problems such as increased heart rate.

The above vignette is an example of a very common issue that a woman might mention to me, as her midwife. It does not mean that Emma has a mental health problem, but it might alert me to spend some time with Emma discussing these issues further and arranging support if necessary.

The midwife and mental health

It is not possible to easily sum up the midwife's role as it is very diverse. As you will have read in other chapters in this book, a midwife examines the woman, provides childbirth education and supports the woman and her family throughout the perinatal period. To do this effectively, the midwife also collaborates with other health and social care professionals to meet the specific needs of mothers today. For example, as well as caring for those women who have a normal pregnancy, birth and postnatal period, the midwife also provides expert care for:

- women with mental health problems;
- women with substance misuse problems;
- teenage mothers;
- women who are socially excluded;
- refugee or asylum seeking women;
- women who experience gender-based violence;
- women from diverse ethnic backgrounds.

(Royal College of Midwives)

The Scottish Executive, Department of Health England, Welsh Assembly Government and Northern Ireland Department of Health, Social Services and Public Safety commissioned Midwifery 2020 (Midwifery 2020, 2010) to explore the scope of midwifery within the U.K. This document reinforced the importance of all midwives in the U.K. as being the lead professional for all healthy women and to coordinate care with key health professionals for those women with more complex needs. Therefore, as you can perhaps see, consideration of the mental health of women in the perinatal period is one aspect of a midwife's varied role in the U.K. However, in light of this U.K.-wide recommendation for midwifery practice, the importance of midwives being involved in women's mental health and well-being within the perinatal period cannot be ignored (Midwifery 2020, 2010), although the nature of this role is often misunderstood and underestimated (Ó Lúanaigh and Carlson 2005; Price 2007). Despite this U.K. recommendation, midwifery education and practice is not the same in all countries as there are differing cultural and professional expectations of a midwife's role. Although I am writing this as a midwife based in Scotland, I have many years' midwifery experience as a clinician and educator on three continents. This has enabled me to recognise that although other countries have similar guidelines for practice, some countries do not embrace the concept of public health as part of the midwife's roles and responsibilities, such as within Europe and the Middle East. Often, midwives' practice in these countries is limited to a specific area of care, such as with women in labour or during the postnatal period. In these situations it is less likely that midwives are aware of the possibilities of a public health role which could allow them to work in a holistic way with women and enable them to address women's mental health needs during this time. Conversely, in Australia I experienced a very proactive approach to perinatal mental health, with many services for women and their families being provided by midwives. As an example of this, I worked in a mother and baby unit within which midwives had an active role caring for the emotional and physical well-being of women, babies and families affected by perinatal mental health problems. Although this topic can perhaps be discussed by considering some issues relevant to perinatal mental health that are pertinent to midwives and their public health role, within just one chapter, I cannot thoroughly explore or justify all aspects of perinatal mental health. Nonetheless, within these limitations I will now attempt to discuss this topic to convey some of the skills required of the midwife. I hope this chapter will be relevant and interesting if you are considering midwifery as a career. This will apply if you are already qualified as an adult nurse or other professional considering a change of career, or those hoping to enter the midwifery profession straight from school or college.

Pregnancy can be a time of psychological change that poses huge challenges and can cause insecurities and anxieties for the woman (Cantwell and Cox 2006). Thus, the common perception in society that being pregnant is a happy, carefree time can be quite the opposite experience for many women; this can further compound their anxieties (Muir 2007). The following excerpt is taken from my own research and is based on a real-life situation (Forrest 2004). This woman was unable to reveal her depression to her husband or her family due to a loss of confidence in herself. She did not want to disappoint them, as she felt they had expectations of her; she therefore continued struggling to keep up the pretence of normality. In doing so she said:

> My husband knew absolutely nothing about it, never knew anything about me going to the doctors. I walked about with dark glasses on constantly. You know, it's funny, but I did believe that 'right well, they can't see me if I put these on' and I really just went about as if I was invisible. Please don't look at me.

The midwife can have a positive impact on the woman just by taking the time to listen. Another example from my study demonstrates how another woman was able to 'open up' because the midwife showed interest in her problems:

> I think initially you can tell when there is somebody there that is sympathetic, that will listen, that may say something when you walk out the door, but at least they are there, they are listening to you, you feel they look interested.

The importance of the midwife as a public health practitioner, and crucial to enhancing overall health, has been clearly shown by research (Ó Lúanaigh and Carlson 2005). Midwifery practice has always engaged public health issues, although this has not always been instantly recognisable. It is important that midwives acknowledge this important aspect of their role and continue to make a significant difference to the public health of women and families. As an example of this, the midwife can provide information, advice and support on issues such as screening, testing, supplementing, for example with folic acid, stopping smoking, breastfeeding promotion and immunisation.

The midwife can also identify the woman with particular needs and develop services to support these. This includes mental health needs. The term perinatal mental health relates to the emotional well-being of parents and infants in the antenatal and postnatal period up to about 1 year after the birth of the baby. An important point to note is that in the majority of women who die by suicide in the perinatal period, serious mood disorder was present (CMACE 2011). Postnatal depression is one aspect of perinatal mental illness that is regarded as being a depressive illness occurring during the first postnatal year. Between 10 and 15 per cent of women suffer postnatal depression (PND) following childbirth (O'Hara and Swain 1996). Until recently, however, depression during pregnancy was not considered (Evans *et al.* 2001), but mental ill health may have been present before the pregnancy commenced or might onset in the antenatal period for a significant proportion of women (Andersson *et al.* 2003). Therefore the term 'perinatal mental health' has allowed a more complete approach to be adopted, which not only considers postnatal problems such as depression and psychosis, but pregnancy-related issues such as anxiety and aspects of how becoming a parent can have an impact on adult mental health. This also addresses existing mental illness and how it can impact on the ability to parent adequately and how it may affect the parent–infant attachment and subsequent relationship. Therefore, the emphasis on providing a more holistic approach to care to minimise negative outcomes within the perinatal mental health period is worth consideration (Austin 2003).

You might wish to consider the following:

Guidance

Our practice as U.K.-based midwives is specifically guided by the Nursing and Midwifery Council (NMC), who produce *Midwives Rules and Standards* (NMC 2013), which must be followed. In relation to perinatal mental health, there are also:

- The recommendations made by publications such as the recent Scottish Intercollegiate Guidelines Network (SIGN) (2012).
- The National Institute for Health and Clinical Excellence (NICE), an independent organisation responsible for providing national guidance on promoting good health and preventing and treating ill health has provided a national clinical guideline for antenatal and postnatal mental health (2007). This guideline (45) specifically only considers the treatment of mental health problems when a pregnancy is being planned, during pregnancy and in the first year after giving birth, therefore is of particular relevance to the work of midwives.
- Additionally, the Confidential Enquiries into Maternal Deaths (CEMD), Why Mother's Die 1997–1999 (2001) Report, and the Confidential Enquiry into Maternal and Child Health (CEMACH) (2004) Why Mothers Die 2000–2002 Report gave midwives information on maternal deaths related to the childbirth

period. This CEMACH report cited psychiatric illness as the most common cause of indirect deaths and the largest cause of maternal deaths overall between 1997 and 2002. More recently, however, the Confidential Enquiry into Maternal and Child Health (CEMACH) Saving Mothers' Lives (2007) and the Centre for Maternal and Child Enquiries (CMACE) (2011) reports have indicated that suicide is no longer the leading cause of indirect maternal deaths during the period 2003–2005 and 2006–2008, respectively. However, it is unclear whether this is as a result of enhanced midwifery care or solely due to an increase in other causes.

This anthology of reports and documents has led to the recognition that perinatal mental illness is a major health issue. These documents also warn against the flippant use of the term postnatal depression (PND), to the detriment of acknowledging a more serious condition. Despite this a lot of focus is still placed on the detection and prevention of PND. The NICE clinical guideline 45 (2007) for antenatal and postnatal mental health recognises that many women have levels of depression, anxiety and distress which may not reach diagnostic criteria for referral to specialist services and it is for this large group of women that midwives can play an important role in offering support. To help with this, the midwife takes a detailed history from each pregnant woman, which includes all obstetric factors, family history and psychosocial issues. It is important for the midwife to remember that normal emotional changes at this time in a woman's life may mask depressive symptoms or be misinterpreted as depression (SIGN 2012). A woman's history and plan of care are recorded in The Scottish Woman-Held Maternity Record (SWHMR). This development by the Scottish government ensures that all women in Scotland have a single unified handheld record during their maternity care (Healthcare Improvement Scotland 2008) and aims to encourage partnership with women and families and continuity of care. A woman's personal and family history of mental illness must be discussed and documented to ensure that the care she requires can be planned. As mentioned before, often the midwife will work with other key health professionals, such as the psychiatric nurse, psychiatrist, health visitor and GP to ensure that the best care possible can be given to meet the woman's individual mental health needs.

The midwife's knowledge and role

To avoid or minimise problems, midwives require an in-depth knowledge of the risk factors for perinatal illness. To do this effectively the midwife must also have good communication and listening skills, to be able to sensitively elicit this information from women and build a trusting, therapeutic relationship. Although it is clear in the literature (NICE 2007) that detecting antenatal risk factors is not in itself predictive of postnatal illness, it can alert midwives to the possibility, and encourage communication between the relevant health care professionals. As directed by NICE clinical guideline 45 (2007), all health care professionals involved in the care of women in the perinatal period should ask two questions to identify possible depression at the time of a woman's first contact with primary care, at her booking visit and in the postnatal period. This emphasises the multi-professional approach to caring for women during this time and can include midwives, obstetricians, health visitors and general practitioners (GPs). The questions recommended to be asked by the NICE guideline are:

1   During the past month, have you often been bothered by feeling down, depressed or hopeless?
2   During the past month, have you often been bothered by having little interest or pleasure in doing things?

A third question should be considered if the woman answers 'yes' to either of the initial questions.

3   Is this something you feel you need or want help with?

Midwives therefore are ideally placed to initiate these questions with women and communicate with the wider multidisciplinary team. Many midwives see women when they attend the GP to have their pregnancy confirmed, or at their booking appointment in the early stages of pregnancy. All midwives have the responsibility to discuss concerns with other colleagues such as midwives, obstetricians, social workers and perinatal mental health practitioners. According to SIGN (2012) the option to admit a woman and her baby to a specialist unit should be available; however, a multi-professional approach to this decision should be made with all members of the team, including family. Many midwives assume particular roles in working closely with perinatal mental health teams. Joint midwifery, obstetric and psychiatric care can then be provided throughout pregnancy, with a plan made for the birth and postnatal care of the woman and the baby. This important liaison role can help to forge better understanding of each professional's contribution and therefore better working relations between different professional groups. The implementation of an integrated care pathway for women, involving midwifery, obstetric and psychiatric care is an example of good practice and collaborative working in which the midwife can be instrumental.

The woman and her family

Additionally it is important for midwives to be aware of the importance of involving women in decision making about their care. This vision is part of the plan for Scotland's maternity services and is outlined in the document, *A Framework for Maternity Services in Scotland* (Scottish Executive 2001). This vision supports the joint working of women, their families and all professionals involved in their care. This involves midwives striving for a particular standard of care to ensure that the needs of women are met. This is particularly relevant not only for the woman but her family. Evidence suggests that perinatal mental health problems in women can result in mental health consequences long term, for the entire family and particularly children (Murray and Cooper 1997; McMahon *et al.* 2001; O'Connor *et al.* 2002). It has also been noted over the last decade and more that many women with perinatal mental health problems often do not seek treatment, due to a perceived stigma of mental health, but also their unrealistic expectations of motherhood (McIntosh 1993). Later studies have shown that detection of PND increases with routine use of a screening tool and therefore suggest that with training, health professionals would have heightened awareness of perinatal mental health problems and could be more able to offer care relevant to women's needs (Buist *et al.* 2006).

The woman's background

When taking a woman's history in relation to perinatal mental health, it is important to know the nature of any past or current illness. This ensures that the best care can be provided and tailored for the individual woman's situation and involves relevant health professionals. For example, the midwife needs to know whether:

- there is any known health problem;
- the woman is currently taking medication;
- she has ever required admission to hospital;
- if so, how long the illness lasted;
- she attends for support and to whom.

It is also important to be able to distinguish any risk factors by gaining information about a family history. The midwife would want to know such things as:

- the nature of the illness;
- that person's relationship to the childbearing woman.

In particular, a close relative with a severe condition, such as bipolar disorder or, possibly, schizophrenia puts a woman at greater risk of perinatal illness. This is most likely to manifest as a psychotic illness, which is a serious episode of mental illness in the postnatal period. Obviously, this could have significant consequences for the woman and the family (Cantwell and Smith 2006).

The midwife should always offer women the opportunity to have 'private time' with her. This would allow discussion of any issues in confidence, without other family members being present. This can pose more of a problem when the community midwife is seeing a woman at home, as there are often family members around. However, the midwife frequently sees the woman at home as part of her community practice. Because of this the midwife becomes intuitive and adaptive if she suspects that there is a problem, but the woman has difficulty discussing it.

The midwife would arrange another visit, when the woman would have more privacy to discuss issues.

The need for 'private time' between the woman and professionals originated with the recognition of the high incidence of gender-based violence (WHO 1997, 2002). Despite the frequency of gender-based violence during the childbearing years (Espinosa and Osborne 2002; Johnson *et al.* 2003) there are still many unanswered questions regarding its precise prevalence. Similarly, risk factors for the woman, her unborn baby and the subsequent consequences of this victimisation are not clear (Jasinski 2004). I have only briefly alluded to this topic within my discussion on perinatal mental health and the role of the midwife. With increasing knowledge, active involvement and as part of their overall public health role, the midwife asks the woman about her risk of harm at home. Midwives will be aware that any woman affected by domestic abuse is at higher risk of developing problems such as depression; she generally lacks support and often feels isolated. As mentioned before, it is crucial for the midwife to recognise the more vulnerable woman. This includes women living with abuse, very young women, homeless women or women from ethnic minorities, especially where there is a language barrier. Often, if social support is lacking, there may be financial and housing difficulties, which can lead to lowered mood or depression (Ó Lúanaigh and Carlson 2005).

After the birth of the baby

The postnatal period is a busy time for the midwife, in that she has to observe both the woman and the baby. The emotional well-being of the woman, and her bonding and attachment with her baby, is just one aspect of midwifery care, as there are many physical checks that should be made. The midwife has to be aware, however, of any factors that potentially put the woman at greater risk of mental illness at this time. For example, it is not always easy to ascertain what a 'difficult birth' is. There are some associations between women who had their first birth by Caesarean, or experienced obstetric complications, and the risk of developing postnatal depression (SIGN 2012). However, the expectation of the individual woman has to be considered, and a woman may report, following what the midwife thinks is a 'normal birth', that it had been a terrible experience for her. This may be a contributing factor or cause of her depression (NICE 2007; SIGN 2012). Often her perception of how well she was supported and involved in the decision-making process will have an influence on her emotional state (NICE 2007; SIGN 2012).

It may be that women who are severely affected by the 'baby blues' are more likely to go on to develop postnatal depression (SIGN 2012). Today, the length of stay in hospital varies greatly. As a result, many women are discharged home by the time any 'blues' become evident. So the community midwife has to be particularly vigilant in her postnatal observations of the woman at home.

In the early postnatal period, the midwife should be alerted to any potential risks of severe mental illness by the woman's antenatal records. In this event, a postnatal plan of action would be in place for the midwife to implement after the woman has given birth. This would be based on the antenatal history, which would have ascertained any past history of severe conditions, such as puerperal psychosis or other mental illness. A known family history of bipolar disorder, or if the woman had been noted to have depression in her pregnancy, would also alert the midwife.

A questionnaire that helps screening for postnatal depression is the Edinburgh Postnatal Depression Scale (EPDS) (Cox and Holden 1994). It is currently used by the health visitor to screen for depression in the postnatal period. It is the role of the midwife, however, to liaise with the GP and health visitor, who will continue care of the woman beyond the midwife's visits.

The midwife in the U.K. is required to care for women until 10 days postnatally. This care normally takes the form of visits to the woman's home which can be tailored to meet the woman and her baby's needs. The midwife can, however, visit for longer if necessary (NMC 2013). The extended role of the midwife in the U.K. is under discussion and the benefits for the midwife and the woman remain uncertain; this is partly because such extended postnatal visiting encroaches on the role of other health professionals. In parts of Europe, postnatal midwives can visit women for a longer period of time, but this can be dependent on health insurance cover and may not be equitable for all women. In Australia, although there has been a growth in postnatal home visits, the majority of care remains as community care, whereby women attend clinics, rather than being seen at home. However, the NMC (2013) is clear within its rules and standards for practice for midwives in the U.K., stating that midwives must only undertake extended roles if they are sufficiently trained to do so. As a midwife with many years of experience working with women and families, together with teaching and research knowledge, I believe the best way forward for women is working as a team to share information effectively. This would enable a seamless service to be provided in order to meet the needs of each individual woman.

In this chapter I have only been able to allude to some of the aspects of perinatal mental health care that the midwife can provide. This service can vary widely depending on the setting, geographical area and country within which the midwife practises, such as hospital, home birth, rural or urban settings. Despite this, each midwife in the U.K. practises with clear guidance from the NMC (2013). There is, however, much scope to develop roles and services dependent on the country or area of practice and the needs of women and their families. If you have a particular interest in perinatal mental health, there are many sources within the literature, journals, textbooks, websites, local and national organisations and government documents to widen your appreciation of this very important topic. We should always remember that a woman's perinatal mental health is of utmost importance, not only to her own well-being, but to that of her children, partner and wider family.

References

Andersson, L., Sundstrom-Poromaa, I., Bixo, M. and Wulff, M. (2003) 'Point prevalence of psychiatric disorders during the second trimester of pregnancy: A population based study'. *American Journal of Obstetrics & Gynecology* 189(1): 148–54.

Austin, M.-P. (2003) 'Perinatal mental health: opportunities and challenges for psychiatry'. *Australasian Psychiatry* 11(4): 399–402.

Buist, A., Condon, J., Brooks, J., Speelman, C., Milgrom, J., Hayes, B., Ellwood, D., Barnett, B., Kowalenko, N., Matthey, S., Austin, M-P. and Bilszta, J. (2006) 'Acceptability of routine screening for perinatal depression'. *Journal of Affective Disorders* 93: 233–237.

Cantwell, R. and Cox, J. (2006) 'Psychiatric disorders in pregnancy and the puerperium'. *Current Obstetrics & Gynaecology* 16: 14–20.

Cantwell, R. and Smith, S. (2006) 'Prediction and prevention of perinatal mental illness'. *Psychiatry* 5(1): 15–21.

Centre for Maternal and Child Enquiries (CMACE) (2011). *Saving Mothers' Lives: Reviewing Maternal Deaths to Make Motherhood Safer: 2006–08*. The Eighth Report on Confidential Enquiries into Maternal Deaths in the United Kingdom. *BJOG* 118(Suppl. 1):1–203.

Confidential Enquiries into Maternal Deaths in the United Kingdom (CEMD) (2001) *Why Mothers Die 1997–1999 Report*. London: RCOG Press.

Confidential Enquiry into Maternal and Child Health (CEMACH) (2004) *Why Mothers Die 2000–2002 Report*: London: RCOG.

Confidential Enquiry into Maternal and Child Health (CEMACH) (2007) *Saving Mothers' Lives: Reviewing Maternal Deaths to Make Motherhood Safer – 2003–2005*. London: RCOG Press.

Cox, J. and Holden, J. (1994) *Perinatal Psychiatry: Use and Misuse of the Edinburgh Postnatal Depression Scale*. London: Gaskell.

Espinosa, L. and Osborne, K. (2002) 'Domestic violence during pregnancy: implications for practice'. *Journal of Midwifery & Women's Health* 47(5): 305–17.

Evans, J., Heron, J., Francomb, H., Oke, S. and Golding, J. (2001) 'Cohort study (ALSPAC) of depressed mood during pregnancy and after childbirth'. *British Medical Journal* 323: 257–60.

Forrest, E. (2004) 'A grounded theory study of services for postnatal depression: women's experiences and perceptions'. Unpublished M.Phil. thesis, Glasgow Caledonian University.

Healthcare Improvement Scotland (2008) Available on line at http://www.healthcare improvementscotland.org. Accessed 21 November 2012.

Jasinski, J.L. (2004) 'Pregnancy and domestic violence: a review of the literature'. *Journal of Trauma Violence & Abuse* 5(1): 47–64.

Johnson, J.K., Haider, F., Ellis, K., Hay, D.M. and Lindow, S.W. (2003) 'The prevalence of domestic violence in pregnant women'. *BJOG: An International Journal of Obstetrics & Gynaecology* 110(3): 272–75.

McMahon, C., Barnett, B., Kowalenko, N., Tennant, C. and Don, N. (2001) 'Postnatal depression, anxiety and unsettled infant behaviour'. *Australian and New Zealand Journal of Psychiatry*, 35: 581–88.

McIntosh, J. (1993) 'Postpartum depression: women's help-seeking behaviour and perceptions of cause'. *Journal of Advanced Nursing* 19: 178–84.

Midwifery 2020 (2010) *Delivering Expectations*. Midwifery 2020 Programme, Cambridge. Available online from: www.midwifery2020.org

Muir, A. (2007) *Overcome Your Postnatal Depression*. London: Hodder Arnold.

Murray, L. and Cooper, P. (1997) 'Postpartum depression and child development'. *Psychological Medicine* 27: 253–60.

National Institute for Health and Clinical Excellence (2007) Guideline 45 *Antenatal and Postnatal Mental Health: Clinical Management and Service Guidance*. London: NICE.

Nursing and Midwifery Council (2013) *Midwives Rules and Standards*. London: NMC.

O'Connor, T., Heron, J., Golding, J., Beveridge, M. and Glover, V. (2002) 'Maternal antenatal anxiety and children's behaviour/emotional problems at 4 years'. *British Journal of Psychiatry* 180: 502–8.

O'Hara, M.W. and Swain, A.M. (1996) 'Rates and risk of postpartum depression – a meta-analysis'. *International Review of Psychiatry* 8: 37–54.

Ó Lúanaigh, P. and Carlson, C. (2005) *Midwifery and Public Health, Future Directions and New Opportunities*. London: Elsevier.

Price, S. (2007) *Mental Health in Pregnancy and Childbirth*. Edinburgh: Elsevier.

Royal College of Midwives. Position Statement on Woman Centred Care. Available on line at http://www.rcm.org.uk/EasysiteWeb/getresource.axd?AssetID=121546 and http://www.rcm.org.uk/college/your-career/want-to-be-a-midwife/

Scottish Executive (2001) *A Framework for Maternity Services in Scotland*. Edinburgh: HMSO.

Scottish Intercollegiate Guidelines Network (2012) SIGN 127 *Management of Perinatal Mood Disorders*. Edinburgh: SIGN Executive.

World Health Organization (1997) *Violence Against Women*. WHO Consultation. Available on line at http://www.who.int/mediacentre/factsheets/fs239/en/. Accessed 22 January, 2013.

World Health Organization (2002) *World Report on Violence and Health*. WHO, Geneva. Available on line at http://www.who.int/topics/violence/en/. Accessed 22 January, 2013.

Commentary

This chapter clearly demonstrates the significance of mental health for the woman, for her baby and for her family. Because of this significance it becomes crucial for the midwife to have a very clear understanding of these issues. Eleanor makes it abundantly apparent, though, that the midwife is far from alone in working with and supporting the woman who has mental health issues. To provide effective help to this woman, her baby and her family, the midwife is required to liaise with colleagues belonging to other disciplines and from different occupational backgrounds.

Thus, mental health conditions provide an excellent example of how the midwife, while invariably individually accountable for her own practice, also needs to be able to function competently and effectively as an active member of a multidisciplinary team. As Eleanor shows, perinatal mental health is in no way an optional extra or an activity to be undertaken if and when time is available. These issues are clearly sufficiently significant to be fundamental to the survival of the woman, and possibly that of her baby as well as the well-being of her family (Oates and Cantwell 2011). It is imperative that these issues are recognised as such by all who are involved with the child-bearing woman.

Reference

Oates, M. and Cantwell, R. (2011) 'Deaths from psychiatric causes', in Centre for Maternal and Child Enquiries (CMACE) *Saving Mothers' Lives: Reviewing Maternal Deaths to Make Motherhood Safer: 2006–08*. The Eighth Report on Confidential Enquiries into Maternal Deaths in the United Kingdom. *BJOG* 118(Suppl. 1):1–203.

6

THE SUPERVISOR OF MIDWIVES AND THE MANAGER

Jean Duerden

There are probably hundreds of different definitions of a supervisor in workplace situations covering many industries from manufacturing to academia. The term supervisor conjures up all sorts of images. It reminds me of a factory foreman supervising all the activity in his department, watching carefully for mistakes or errors in the processes and ensuring that a perfect product emerges at the end of the conveyor belt. In some ways, I suppose this could be quite a good analogy for midwifery; the supervisor of midwives watching carefully, seeing that no mistakes are made and that only the highest standard of midwifery care is offered in her department, and ensuring that the end result is the birth of a healthy baby with no ill effects on the mother. This does, however, sound somewhat inspectoral and sadly some midwives might see supervision in that light rather than in the supportive sense that it should be perceived. I hope to change any perception of punitive supervision to one of supportive supervision during this chapter.

If you are reading this book as a midwife for reflective purposes, deciding whether to stay in midwifery, you might have your own story to tell about supervision. I would hope that this story is a positive one, describing a supportive supervisor of midwives. In which case there may be little to tell as we sometimes forget the good things that happen to us. Support from a supervisor of midwives can be quite discreet and so much a part of everyday midwifery that it doesn't always provide a significant memory when having a conversation. It appears, though, that our minds are tuned to recalling negative rather than positive events. It's a bit like newspapers only printing the bad news, so if your supervision experience was particularly difficult and badly handled you will be more anxious to share your story and you may have turned first to this chapter to explore the supervision of midwives more thoroughly.

The current shortage of midwives means that those working in busy maternity units have to make critical decisions when prioritising their work loads. No one can forecast the future and, despite years of research, determining how quickly labour will advance is an imperfect science, despite the fact that many women think midwives have the answer and will constantly ask for an estimate of how long until their baby is born. As a consequence, it takes a lot of experience, and even more good luck, to determine what care and attention women need in labour. We all know that in the ideal world there would be one midwife caring solely for one woman in labour but, as the introduction to this book clearly states, we are not living in an ideal world but within NHS constraints. The labour ward co-ordinator has one of the most difficult jobs in allocating staff on each shift. I am sure that experienced midwives reading this book can relate to the incident that I will describe through a short vignette, and for those considering a career in midwifery you can learn how an incident in a maternity unit was successfully managed through supervision.

VIGNETTE

The maternity unit was extremely busy. It was impossible to give one-on-one care to every woman in labour. Jen, a newly qualified midwife, was caring for two women on her night shift. It seemed that one of the women she was caring for, Amy, was a long way off giving birth so she tried to focus her attention on Lizzie whose birth appeared more imminent. Jen checked that Amy was comfortable and that her partner Andy was OK. Unfortunately, the CTG trace in Lizzie's room showed signs of fetal distress so Jen called the registrar and Lizzie was rapidly taken to theatre for Caesarean section.

It was over an hour before Jen got back to Amy and Andy's room where Amy was now in advanced labour. They were both very anxious as no one had been in to see them. Because no one had been observing Amy, there were no records of maternal observation and no record of the fetal monitoring or contractions as there was no paper left in the CTG monitor; it had run out during Jen's absence. Jen realised with horror that she had not briefed the labour ward co-ordinator when she was leaving the ward or told her that Amy would need regular checking. Although she should have been supernumerary, the busyness of the labour ward that night had meant that the co-ordinator was also caring for women in labour.

After Jen's return, Amy progressed to give birth to a normal healthy baby but Jen knew she had not ensured that Amy had received continuing care during her labour and what might have been haunted her and caused concern for the labour ward co-ordinator.

Making a mistake is punishment enough for any midwife, so the supervisor of midwives realises that taking punitive action is neither fair nor appropriate. So let's see how this situation was handled by Sue, the supervisor of midwives.

VIGNETTE

Sue learned about the incident when Jen phoned her soon afterwards. Jen hoped that by contacting Sue as soon as possible after the incident she would get the support she anticipated; which she did.

Sue knew that the outcome of this incident could have been very different and, in her long experience as a supervisor of midwives, she had dealt with a similar incident where the baby had been badly affected. In the event of a serious incident involving a midwife, a supervisor of midwives will undertake a supervisory enquiry on behalf of the Local Supervising Authority (LSA). On this occasion there was no LSA enquiry but the labour ward co-ordinator met with Jen and Sue to talk through the incident. Sue had to console Jen as it was a very difficult meeting and she felt quite wretched and devastated by her mistake that could have had such far-reaching consequences.

Sue had to decide how best Jen could be helped. She knew that to restore Jen's confidence she would need local action under the supervision of her named supervisor using a learning contract. Local action under the supervision of her named supervisor is a time-limited programme of working with the support of a supervisor but not under direct supervision. The midwife concerned meets regularly with her supervisor during the programme to discuss the women she has cared for and the care she gave. She will also discuss the progress she is making with her learning contract. In this case, the learning contract involved a record-keeping programme and CTG update with a mentor for Jen to assist her with this. Sue asked Jen who she thought was the best person to be her mentor; it needed to be a midwife who she respected and had good knowledge of record-keeping requirements and CTG. Jen chose the practice development midwife who was delighted to help. The time limit for achieving all the aims of the learning contract was 4 weeks and, with Sue's support, Jen achieved all the aims and was able to confidently continue working on the labour ward.

Confidentiality was maintained throughout this process with only Sue and the mentor being aware that Jen was working through a learning contract. The regular meetings gave Jen a chance to discuss with Sue how she had come to terms with her error and how she felt she had learned, in fact benefited, from this. She was able to demonstrate a new confidence from her improved knowledge. The practice development midwife had completed CTG assessment with Jen and they were both pleased with the results. Jen's record keeping improved as did her understanding of the need for accurate, contemporaneous records.

Sue didn't just leave Jen to it at the end of the learning contract, but she made regular informal contact to ensure that Jen was happy and confident in her work and knew that she was there if needed.

I hope that this vignette has demonstrated the positive response that supervision provides in the twenty-first century and how the supervisor of midwives is there for the midwife through thick and thin. Sadly there will be circumstances where the outcome is not so good and instead of 'what might have been' haunting Jen it could have been 'what has been'. How critical incidents are managed is described later in this chapter, but no matter what level of incident, the named supervisor of midwives is there to provide support for every midwife on her caseload.

Supervisors of midwives are not there just for the bad days. There are also plenty of examples of supervisors responding positively to midwives when they have done well such as through new academic achievement or promotion. The supervisor is there to enjoy those good moments as well as the more difficult times.

The introduction to this book abandons any rose-tinted spectacles and describes vividly how midwifery has changed and with greater rapidity over recent years. Struggling within this changing profession, newly qualified midwives and those with long experience can feel very isolated, so it is essential to have a good relationship with your supervisor of midwives from the start to build up the belief in supervision that is needed to make it work. Sue, in the vignette, had made contact with Jen as soon as she started work at the maternity unit when she was told that Jen had been allocated to her as a supervisor of midwives. Sue knew Jen when she was a student midwife and was delighted when Jen had chosen her as her supervisor. They were slowly building a good relationship and Sue's aim was that this would be based on mutual respect.

Having an element of choice in the allocation of midwife to supervisor is essential, and that can be both ways, with the midwife choosing her supervisor and the supervisor choosing her supervisees. Usually, the midwife is invited to select three supervisors she would be happy to have as her named supervisor of midwives and the supervisor also has the opportunity to say no if her list is already full or she would not feel confident with that midwife–supervisor relationship. You must not lose sight of the fact that the supervisor is also a practising midwife who will also experience the highs and lows of midwifery practice and be affected by the same constraints imposed by the changing NHS. With the increase of specialist roles for midwives you could feel that a supervisor of midwives working in a different specialism from you will not understand your personal area of work or have the appropriate level of expertise, but supervision is not about expert knowledge in every area of practice but understanding the basic needs of midwives, their hopes and plans for the future, the professional development needed to achieve their goals and showing empathy when they find practice increasingly stressful.

Investigating critical incidents is not easy, no matter what the outcome. A supervisor of midwives is well aware that, despite the blame culture that we appear to live in, no one deliberately tries to harm women or babies; perhaps the infamous nurse Beverley Allitt was the exception (Appleyard 1994). Similarly no midwife is a fool; how could a fool qualify as a midwife? This means the supervisor's starting point in any supervisory enquiry must be 'what are the extenuating circumstances?'

Following a serious critical incident, there will inevitably be a management enquiry commissioned by the Trust through their risk management policy, but the supervisor acts independently of the Trust and on behalf of the LSA. It is not appropriate for the named supervisor of midwives to undertake this enquiry as she needs to be available to support the midwife and listen to her account of events. Another supervisor of midwives will be asked to undertake the supervisory enquiry on behalf of the LSA. The best approach is for the supervisor to get everyone together, meeting with all the midwives involved. It is very important to get the whole story from everyone at the same time so that each midwife knows what happened when they were not in the birthing room. It helps everyone to get the true picture and to understand how the event developed.

Maintaining confidentiality is not easy when it is determined that an LSA practice programme, rather than local action is needed. When an LSA practice programme is advocated the midwife concerned must work all the time in a supernumerary capacity under the direct supervision of a clinical mentor for a prescribed amount of time, with academic assessment by a midwifery lecturer. This might seem harsh, but after a very serious incident the midwife's confidence can be badly knocked and she will feel more confident working with a supervisor. Similarly, the supervisor needs to know that the midwife can practise safely and the public need assurance of the safety of midwifery practice.

An old fashioned response to a labour ward incident in many hospitals might have been to remove the midwife from the labour ward to work in the postnatal ward. But, just as getting back on your bike after falling off is the best approach, it is best to continue working in the same area. You cannot learn about best care in labour on a postnatal ward.

The vignette describes a hospital incident but it could just as easily have been a birth centre or home birth situation. Midwives value their role as autonomous practitioners and being able to work independently of medical staff in the home birth situation emphasises this more than any other. It can be quite daunting for a midwife used to having plenty of people around in the hospital, especially the first home birth. There is a supervisor of midwives available 24/7 in every area, so a midwife attending a home birth can contact the supervisor at any time for advice and a second opinion. Just having someone to bounce ideas off, especially when you are tired and/or stressed, can make a huge difference and this kind of support is much appreciated by the midwife attending a home birth. Independent midwives who, whilst they are still able to practise, work mostly in the home environment also appreciate having a supervisor of midwives at the other end of the telephone.

I deliberately chose a newly qualified midwife to use as an example in the vignette. The sudden change from student to qualified midwife has been mentioned elsewhere in this book but deserves further mention in a chapter on supervision. Although we welcome the autonomy of the midwife's role, it is the most challenging aspect of midwifery for the newly registered. Having, as a student, trained in a position of direct supervision and mentorship, the newly qualified midwife is expected to be capable of autonomous decision making overnight. Many have described this experience as being 'thrown into the lions' den'. Unfortunately, reduced staffing levels in many maternity units have led to newly qualified midwives being counted as pairs of hands on an understaffed shift, prohibiting well-managed preceptorship.

The current recommendation from the NMC (Nursing amd Midwifery Council) is for new registrants to have protected learning time in the first year of qualified practice with access to and regular meetings with a preceptor (NMC 2008). Not many midwives can recount working alongside their preceptor on every shift in their first few weeks in post and sometimes the off-duty patterns of preceptor and newly qualified midwife (NQM) are not compatible. However, NQMs can seek support and advice from the supervisor of midwives if this situation arises, as it leaves the NQM and women in her care vulnerable until the midwife has confidence through consolidating her experience.

The principle of preceptorship is to provide support and guidance for new registrants and enable them to make the transition from student to accountable practitioner (NMC 2006a). The NQM should thus have protected learning time for at least 4 months. The preceptor provides positive feedback on good performance and honest and objective feedback where performance could be improved, at the same time as facilitating new knowledge and skills. This is a tall order for any midwife working in a busy unit and on different shifts from the new registrant. With careful planning, however, it can work well and part of the supervisor of midwives' first meeting with the NQM will be to check that a preceptor has been allocated and that the relationship is working.

All this might seem an idyllic presentation of supervision but this is how supervision can and does work. There will always be exceptions, though, especially where different personalities are involved. Each individual supervisor of midwives will have different characteristics that will make her into a different kind of supervisor, but the guidance for supervisors is clear and easily available through many of the NMC publications, particularly the 'Midwives rules and standards 2012 (NMC 2012) introduced in 2013, and 'Standards for the preparation and practice of supervisors of midwives' (NMC 2006b). There is also a lot of helpful material for midwives on how to make the most of supervision in 'Modern Supervision in Action – a practical guide for midwives' (LSAMO/NMC 2009).

Supervision has a very long history, being first introduced in 1902 in England. More than 110 years later it continues to work effectively; limiting the number of midwives being referred to the NMC. It must, however, be used appropriately to be effective and it relies on a good relationship between the midwife and supervisor of midwives. It goes without saying that the supervision offered in 1902 is a far cry from that practised in 2014. The original style was very inspectoral – and with good reason. We all remember Charles Dickens' apocryphal character Sairey Gamp in Martin Chuzzlewit, first published in 1844 (Dickens 1994). One cannot be sure that Dickens based her on a real life midwife but 60 years later there were still some very unsavoury midwives around and their inspection and regulation improved standards of care for women and babies. The recent BBC TV series *Call the Midwife* brilliantly demonstrated the plight of midwives working in very restricted circumstances, challenging on-call rotas leading to exhaustion as well as the daily dangers of travelling alone in London's dockland. There was no clear identification of a supervisor of midwives but the support provided by the sister in charge at Nonnatus house, Sister Julienne, to me is the epitome of the ideal supervisor of midwives. The programme has led to a 17 per cent increase in applications for midwifery training (Furness 2013) causing problems for UCAS and huge disappointment to many keen would-be midwives.

For over 110 years, supervisors of midwives have been charged with protecting the public. Within recent years, however, the emphasis of the role has changed and supporting midwives is much more to the fore. It stands to reason though, that if a midwife is supported she is less likely to perform sub-optimally and more likely to seek advice when she is unsure about a situation and ask for help when needed (Page 2010). Having a supervisor, perhaps like Sister Julienne, who is approachable and wise, makes seeking help so much easier.

The supervisor of midwives is also there for women but it has always proved difficult to get this message across to women whose first contact is with the midwife. They are unlikely to have contact, or need contact, with a supervisor of midwives if all goes well in their care. Sadly, it is usually only when something goes wrong or when her needs are not being met that a woman learns about the role of the supervisor. To address this, the NMC has published a revised booklet called *Supervisors of Midwives: How can they help you?* (NMC 2010). The booklet explains who supervisors of midwives are and what they can do for you, such as providing advice about options for care and listening to concerns about care received.

Whether a midwife is newly qualified or has been practising for many years, she will still value her annual review with her supervisor of midwives. This is protected, personal time for the midwife for a reflective review of her midwifery practice during the previous year. She can discuss her aspirations for the coming year and seek the supervisor's support in providing learning opportunities to achieve those aspirations. Any concerns about practice can be discussed in this confidential arena secure in the knowledge that the supervisor is in a position to offer support and guidance and take action where needed.

It is not intended to give the impression that midwives should be totally dependent on their supervisor of midwives. Far from it, over-dependence would be a trial to the supervisor and would not assist the midwife in her personal development. Ideally, the supervisory relationship should be one of empowerment and this can only be achieved if there is respect for supervision and the supervisor.

The supervisor of midwives is a practising midwife herself and, although many midwifery managers are supervisors of midwives, the majority are clinical midwives. This means that the supervisors have their own dilemmas in clinical practice and need the help and support of their own supervisors. Supervision is part of the wonderful chain of 'caring for the carers' within midwifery. The mother cares for her baby, the midwife cares for the mother, the supervisor of midwives cares for the midwife and the supervisor's supervisor of midwives cares for her.

The LSA midwifery officer (LSAMO) is responsible for the supervision of midwives within her area. There are 15 LSAMOs in the UK covering large areas. They visit each Trust annually to monitor the supervision and standards of midwifery and supervisory practice and in turn the NMC audits each LSA on a 3-year cycle. Despite covering such huge areas with thousands of midwives notifying their intention to practise to each officer, they can still be approached by individual midwives or parents if they feel that supervision is not being carried out appropriately in their area or if there are any concerns about midwifery practice that the caller believes are not being addressed. The LSAMO will then investigate accordingly.

Even if a supervisor of midwives is also a manager, supervision and management are different and the two roles have to be clearly defined, although this may not always be easy for the supervisor/manager concerned. When responding to incidents, supervisor/managers have to make it clear in which capacity they are acting. The manager of the area where an incident has taken place has to abdicate all supervisory responsibilities in order to focus on risk management for the Trust; another supervisor will be asked to carry out the supervisory enquiry. For example, in the vignette, the manager of the labour ward would act on behalf of the Trust to consider the risk management aspects of the incident. Obviously the staffing levels on the unit had a part to play in what happened and that is certainly a management issue.

Supervision, as any aspect of any profession, may have had its criticisms. This could perhaps be due to misunderstanding of the role. The LSAMO/NMC publication aims to resolve those misunderstandings (LSAMO/NMC 2009). One of those misunderstandings is regarding the LSAMO having the power to suspend a midwife from practice. This is not something that happens frequently and is also confused with suspension from duty. The former can only be done by an LSAMO and refers to preventing a midwife from practising anywhere, whilst the latter refers to a Trust preventing a midwife from working in the Trust pending a disciplinary hearing. These powers are needed in order to protect the public, but are rarely used.

Other misunderstandings are that supervisors are there to inspect and criticise. It is interesting that early in the last century the Central Midwives Board advised that the supervisor of midwives should be a 'friend and counsellor' rather than a 'relentless critic' (MoH 1937). Supervisors are certainly expected to monitor midwifery practice but criticism should be constructive and helpful and the response to any incident should be proactive rather than reactive and punitive. That proactive response must also be appropriate, hence the two levels of response to serious incidents: local action under the supervision of a named supervisor or an LSA practice programme. The NMC believes there is evidence to demonstrate that effective supervision of midwives can successfully re-empower those midwives who have been on programmes put in place by LSAs (NMC 2013).

The majority of supervision is undertaken without either action and I hope I have described how it can have a very positive effect on midwifery practice and midwives.

Acknowledgement

Carol Paeglis was my successor as LSAMO for Yorkshire and she has kindly proofread and amended my chapter to ensure it is up-to-date and relevant. I am very grateful to her for this support.

References

Appleyard, W.J. (1994) 'Murder in the NHS'. *British Medical Journal* 308: 287–8 (29 January).

Dickens, C. (1994) *Martin Chuzzlewit*. Ware: Wordsworth Editions Ltd.

Furness, H. (2013) '*Call the Midwife* sparks surge in student applications'. *Daily Telegraph*, 10 January.

LSAMO/NMC Midwifery Officers National (UK) Forum & Nursing and Midwifery Council (2009) *Modern Supervision in Action – A Practical Guide for Midwives*. London: Nursing and Midwifery Council.

MoH (1937) *Circular 1620 Supervision of Midwives*. Ministry of Health.

NMC (2006a) *Circular 21/2006 Preceptorship Guidelines*. London: Nursing and Midwifery Council.

NMC (2006b) *Standards for the Preparation and Practice of Supervisors of Midwives*. London: Nursing and Midwifery Council.

NMC (2008) *Standards to Support Learning and Assessment in Practice*. London: Nursing and Midwifery Council.

NMC (2010) *Supervisors of Midwives: How Can They Help You?* London: Nursing and Midwifery Council.

NMC (2012) *Midwives Rules and Standards 2012*. London: Nursing and Midwifery Council.

NMC (2013) *Supervision, Support and Safety. Report of the Quality Assurance of Local Supervising Authorities 2011–2012*. London: Nursing and Midwifery Council.

Page, M. (2010) 'Embracing uncertainty: supporting normal birth'. Unpublished PhD thesis, Queen Margaret University.

Commentary

In this chapter Jean begins by outlining a scenario with potentially disastrous consequences. Fortunately the occasion she describes had a happy ending but it has implications for clinicians, managers and supervisors. It might be asked 'What is the difference between management and supervision'? Jean seeks to forestall this question by providing a robust definition of supervision and making a clear differentiation between supervision and management in midwifery. For those midwives in practice elsewhere than in the United Kingdom, further questions may come to mind as to its necessity, as it is not something that is well known beyond that country. Other countries such as New Zealand, for instance, have robust peer review processes of all midwives as an alternative but in the UK the statutory requirement for supervision has been in place for over 100 years. As Jean explains, not only has the aim changed but also the models of supervision employed to achieve it.

Midwifery of course is not the only health profession to utilise a process of supervision but in mental health nursing, which practises supervision internationally, the approach adopted is more focused on regular meetings between small groups of nurses and one supervisor (White & Winstanley 2010), while in midwifery the process is more fluid.

In her chapter Jean has shown how the process can be initiated from any of the parties involved. Following the incident described in the vignette the process was initiated by the midwife herself, who as a newly qualified midwife was seeking (and receiving) support from her supervisor. A planned programme of action clearly led to positive results for all concerned. However, midwifery supervision has not always been so supportive, as Kirkham & Stapleton (2000) reported from the large grounded theory study they carried out in England. The authors of this study clearly highlighted the need for change within the National Health Service and just as clearly Jean's chapter portrays one area's response to those calls for change and the supportive atmosphere that has resulted.

References

Kirkham, M. and Stapleton, H. (2000) 'Midwives' support needs as childbirth changes'. *Journal of Advanced Nursing* 32(2): 465–72.

White, E. and Winstanley, J. (2010) 'A randomised controlled trial of clinical supervision: selected findings from a novel Australian attempt to establish the evidence base for causal relationships with quality of care and patient outcomes, as an informed contribution to mental health nursing practice development'. *Journal of Research in Nursing* 15: 151–67.

7

THE ACADEMIC MIDWIFE

Rosemary Mander

In this chapter I plan to explore the significance of midwifery education and the extent to which achieving the education of the midwifery student impinges on the academic midwife who is charged with, *inter alia*, ensuring that the midwife who practises as such has been suitably prepared. In order to achieve this aim, first I consider some of the terminology which may be used and how it may affect the academic midwife. Because it occupies so much of her working life, next I outline relevant issues relating to developments in midwifery education. Third, a particular aspect of this midwife's role has assumed immense importance and so I need to address the problem of clinical credibility, which features in my vignette. Finally, I consider two admittedly political aspects; these are the pursuit of academic freedom and the 'two camps' phenomenon with the academic midwife's ability to survive with a foot in both.

The term 'academic' is sometimes used disparagingly as it may carry negative connotations. This is because it bears an aura of being detached from reality, bringing to mind elitist accusations associated with ivory towers. For this reason it may be helpful to consider what 'academic' actually means, before contemplating my role. First, to be a teacher or lecturer is one aspect. Second, being research active is fundamentally important to the academic, but I have to avoid duplication of Ans Luyben's excellent explication of that role (see Chapter 8). Last but not least, the academic midwife's administrative functions are manifold and variably satisfying, so I will refrain from giving them too much attention.

Regarding the A-word, a term which may be preferable, although it tends to be used less frequently is 'scholar', which an online dictionary defines as a 'learned person, educated person; expert in a particular field' (Dictionarist 2013). This definition is useful because it shows the breadth of what being a scholar or an academic is all about. The same dictionary interestingly includes a reference to 'theory', which may be considered less appropriate, especially for a practice discipline (see Introduction). In this chapter I will be further teasing out the various aspects of this role and addressing both the positive and other aspects.

Defining the term is necessary, largely because of the lack of written material focusing on the academic midwife, as identified by a search engine. The work of Claire MacKenzie (2004) in Australia is an important exception to this observation. Her writing has to be contrasted with the enthusiasm with which certain, well-defined, groups of nurses write about academic nursing (for example, Thompson & Watson 2001, 2006; Laiho 2010).

The role of the academic midwife as a teacher tends to be the aspect which comes most easily to mind; it is the education, and associated socialisation, of midwifery students which ensures a suitable foundation for midwives and midwifery care (Benoit *et al.* 2001). Midwifery education in the UK and other countries has undergone momentous developments in the latter part of the twentieth century and has assumed a dynamism which is likely to continue. These developments mean that midwifery education and the midwifery student have changed out of all recognition. The result is that the midwife is now of a 'different breed' (Bower 2002:150) when compared with the midwife who was educated before these developments were implemented.

The largest component of the role of the midwife educationalist is usually the pre-registration midwifery programme, which is university-based and avoids the medical orientation of a pre-requisite nursing qualification. That the midwife does not bring to her practice the baggage of a nursing education is thought to increase the likelihood of more autonomous practice (Benoit *et al.* 2001:356). Some practitioners consider, however, that a university education carries a danger of the midwife becoming too theoretically, rather than clinically, focused (Hunt 1996); although educationalists tend to perceive the benefits of a sound university education to benefit the care of the childbearing woman (Alexander 1994).

The pre-registration programme will feature formal face-to-face, as well as small-group and virtual or online, teaching. The preparation of online and other materials is time consuming and needs to demonstrate a research basis and, it is to be hoped, activity. In relation to the student's vitally important clinical learning experience, clinical mentorship preparation and support are intended to ensure an appropriate learning environment. The assessment, marking and feedback on the student's work are crucial, particularly for the student, as is student support, both pre-admission and on-programme, together with follow-up activities, such as employment references. Because of the dynamic nature of midwifery education, preparation of new programmes and curriculum development with other members of the midwifery education team, and possibly other disciplines if shared learning is offered, feature prominently. As in any collegial environment, peer support, particularly for less-experienced colleagues, is time well spent. In addition, super-vision and other support are offered to postgraduate and research students.

In view of academics employed in higher education institutions (HEIs) being involved with teaching, administration and research, they contemplate long and hard how to spread themselves thinly enough to be able to cover all three aspects.

Sometimes staff are employed, probably at a lower grade, to undertake only teaching; this is a strategy which clearly reflects the relatively low priority attached by universities to their teaching obligations. It may be argued, however, that in some of the newer universities, teaching is prioritised at the expense of staff undertaking other activities, such as research.

Because of the nature of midwifery as a practice discipline, these three domains, which in themselves are challenging, have been extended. At the behest of a previous statutory regulatory body, *The Future of Professional Practice* (UKCC 1994) recommended the inclusion of a fourth, clinical, component. Thus, midwifery and nursing educationalists became required to develop clinical experience and expertise which is up to date, relevant and research based. This requirement may be said to create a new triad of the traditional '3Rs'. For the academic midwife, to 'research' and 'writing', has been added the need to move away from the 'ivory tower' mind-set by being firmly grounded in 'reality'.

This extension of the academic role has become transformed by various pundits and authorities, not to mention midwife academics themselves, into the much sought-after, but seriously evasive, phenomenon which goes by the name of 'clinical credibility'. For these staff, many of whom were in the process of being transferred to a very different employment culture, the bar was being raised to an unrealistically high level. The difficulties of being 'all things to all people' were recognised at the time (Hunt 1998; Jackson 1999) and have continued to be seen as somewhat problematical (NMC 2010).

The credibility of the academic midwife in the clinical area may not be easily distinguished from her clinical competence. The significance of these twin goals, however, relates to the well-known problem of a discrepancy between midwifery education and the reality of clinical practice, widely known as the 'theory–practice gap'. Bridging this gap, it tends to be assumed, will ensure an educational programme which will increase the likelihood of the practitioner being 'fit for practice' (UKCC 2001). The way in which the twin goals of clinical credibility and competence are achieved is even more challenging, as I have made apparent in my vignette (below).

The lack of attention given by midwives to the problem of clinical credibility was the stimulus for a small study by Carol Hindley (1997). This study demonstrated academic staff and midwifery students' enthusiasm, but clinical staff's misgivings about teaching staff involvement. The findings of an up-to-date study by Val Collington and her colleagues (2012), were more authoritative, but were also disappointingly consistent with Hindley's. The recent study indicates that while clinical practice and credibility are undertaken and sought, respectively, to ensure effective midwifery education, those who actively participate in academic clinical practice view any benefits as more restricted, personal and direct. This salutary finding resonates with the discomfortingly probing question articulated by Heather Bower about the limited credibility of the midwife lecturer in either the clinical area or the higher education setting (2002:161). Such lack of credibility may be compared unfavourably with medical education, which exudes confidence in both settings.

In the same way as clinical freedom is assiduously claimed and vociferously defended by certain health care professionals, so academic freedom is a phrase which trips off the tongue, all too often unthinkingly. It is a term which raises visions of a generally easy life in the form of long sunshiny sabbaticals and a jet-setting lifestyle. In my experience, sabbatical or study leave has been changed from being an employment right to becoming a hard-won privilege. And the jet-setting has, for me at least, featured proofreading manuscripts or marking course work in uncongenial environments such as departure lounges and replacement buses.

As universities have been rationalised and commercial pressures applied, staff–student ratios have deteriorated and the notion of academic freedom has receded with it. With that proviso, however, innovation is generally applauded in teaching, publication and research. I have enjoyed the ability to introduce novel forms of education and practice with the input, and sometimes support, of clinical colleagues (Mander 1989, 1992; Mander *et al.* 2010).

As is so often the case, though, academic freedom can be a mixed blessing. The academic's ability to assume control of their working life may be real enough, within the organisational constraints mentioned already. The nature of the academic environment, though, needs to be taken into account. The institution, especially in the older universities, demonstrates a deeply masculinised and patriarchal orientation, which assumes that all members of staff have the liberty to work freely, unfettered by the demands of domestic and social encumbrances. For many, especially women academics, it is necessary to accept these ground rules if there is any intention to make progress in an academic career. This is likely to mean that difficult decisions need to be made. The result is that there is a tendency in such a masculinised milieu to resort to a workaholic approach, with little, if any, consideration for the work/life balance. It is for these reasons that academic freedom should more accurately be regarded as something of a double-edged sword.

As would be widely expected, the role of the midwife academic, like other teaching personnel in HEIs, is focused mainly on teaching, in addition to other aspects of the midwifery student's learning experience. It may be, however, that midwife academics are more conscientious in these matters than their higher education colleagues. This observation may relate to the precise midwifery focus on the welfare of the woman and her baby, compared with a less direct focus of concern in more theoretical disciplines. The midwifery teaching remit extends to include a range of political and policy developments which influence the midwifery student, the student's learning experience and eventual practice and, ultimately, the care of the childbearing woman and her baby (Bower 2002). I would argue, therefore, that the midwife educationalist has, like her counterpart in practice is 'with woman', the role of being 'with student'. In this way the midwife academic is perfectly positioned to serve as a scholarly role model.

For the academic working in another field the priorities are likely to be different. A more masculine approach to education is likely to result in the student being left to their own devices to make the most of the learning opportunities which they are able to identify. In this way the academic, with reduced teaching and student demands, is able to take time to focus on other activities. These are likely to include pursuits which serve to earn, for the individual, the department and the institution, 'brownie points' in the form of promotion, research income and peer recognition. Thus, it is starting to become apparent that the midwife educationalist may encounter a culture of teaching in a university setting which is different from that anticipated, based on previous experience in health care settings (Kenny *et al.* 2004). And the midwife academic may find that efforts to comply with the UKCC recommendation of clinical credibility are met, not with enthusiastic admiration, but with blank bemusement that the groundrules have not been identified, let alone pursued. Thus, the midwife academic may find that they are in the disconcerting position of struggling to seek out, locate and then aim for the goal posts.

Writing in the context of nursing in England, Gerard Kenny and his colleagues probe some of the elephant traps which beset the novice entering academe (2004). In addition to the unanticipated teaching orientation mentioned already, Kenny *et al.* highlight the gender bias which is inherent in masculinised and possibly patriarchal HEIs, observing that:

> Female academics may need to work on implicit gender relations and structural oppression to make them explicit and so they can be engaged with and challenged.
>
> *(Kenny et al. 2004:633)*

These authors comment on the effect on the novice academic's previously acquired professional values of the organisational constraints integral to HEIs. For this reason, ethical problems inevitably arise through professional ideals being compromised by the demands of oversized and hierarchical institutions, whose flexibility is curtailed by an ever-increasing burden of commercialisation. It becomes apparent that Kenny and his colleagues are concerned that the power associated with oppressive educational structures may limit the academic's autonomy and reflective self-awareness. Their solution is to resort to increasingly manipulative political activity.

This scathing criticism by Kenny and his colleagues of the culture of HEIs only serves to clarify the difficulties which are encountered by the midwife academic. Encouraged by statutory and other bodies to ensure the relevance of teaching to practice, the midwife academic must seek to maintain credibility in not only the clinical but also the academic sphere. This person is faced with the problems of moving between and functioning at an authoritative level within the two worlds which are the clinical area and the educational institution. There is a constant adjustment and readjustment of orientation and stance in order to sustain and demonstrate the degree of knowledge and expertise needed to function optimally in both sites. Thus, the academic midwife, unlike her midwifery and her university peers, endeavours to retain an appropriate standing; this is while maintaining a foot in both camps, neither of which comprehends the nature of academic midwifery and the challenges involved.

This slightly bleak picture, however, may be something of an overstatement. While the differences between the two spheres clearly exist, universities and clinical settings have much in common. This means that the problems which I have outlined may not be as real as apparent. The crucially important commonalities are found in the two sectors, health care and higher education. These organisations share features in common because they are both male-dominated hierarchical institutions. Cecilia Benoit and her multinational colleagues' critique of the UK National Health Service, featuring 'cost constraints, staff shortages, policies that are not family-friendly, and unequal opportunities' (2001:357), may also be applied most pertinently to UK HEIs. Both sectors have been reduced by governmental stringencies to assuming basically commercial approaches to what would otherwise be altruistic activities. For this reason I am arguing that astute political manoeuvrability is an essential prerequisite for a person contemplating a career in midwifery or higher education or combining the two to become an academic midwife.

VIGNETTE

I've changed the ordinary clothes which I wear as an academic to put on one of those white things. I am now entering the maternity unit as a midwife 'without status', as my honorary contract puts it. Each time I walk along this corridor a flood of diverse emotions engulfs me. On the one hand, I feel misgivings at the false security which donning a uniform offers. This bogus security reminds me of the anxieties which the childbearing woman must experience when walking the same corridor if she is to be admitted. At the forefront of my mind are the perceptions of my midwife colleagues who, knowing that I am employed in a university, may harbour unrealistically high expectations of my knowledge and expertise. More disconcertingly I fear that the clinical credibility for which I strive will be exposed as a fraudulent façade and that this exposure will involve damage to the women to whom I am assigned to provide care.

Amid this familiar maelstrom of the mind, I see walking towards me a figure I recognise. It is Zoë (not her real name), who had been an undergraduate nursing student a few years previously. She was one of those challenging students who needed to know the source of and reference for every observation or statement. In a nutshell she was bright and stimulating, but not easy.

It had not surprised me when she told me, just before her nursing graduation, that she did not accept the picture which I painted of childbearing. She had continued by saying that reading and research were a pointless waste of time and money, and that the only way to learn about maternity was by doing what she planned – this was by having her own baby. 'That's really good', I had managed to articulate through gritted teeth. 'Keep in touch.'

Now here she is walking out of the maternity unit, dressed as a midwife, with a broad smile. She tells me that she's completed her midwifery programme; she has come back to a job on the combined ante/postnatal ward, while she is trying to find a post in the community. And she is loving being a midwife.

She is interested to know what I am doing and why I am here. I explain my clinical hours and how they are of value in informing my academic role. I see the penny drop and the pieces fall into place.

'Right', she says slowly, thoughtfully and, it seems to me, perhaps a little reluctantly. 'Now I understand.'

'By the way', she releases her parting shot. 'You were pretty well right in all that you said to us.'

References

Alexander, J. (1994) 'Degree of difference'. *Modern Midwife* 4(8): 24–6.

Benoit, C., Davis-Floyd, R., van Teijlingen, E., Sandall, J. and Miller, J. (2001) 'Designing midwives: a comparison of educational models', in R. DeVries (sic), C. Benoit, E. van Teijlingen and S. Wrede (eds), *Birth by Design: Pregnancy, Maternity Care, and Midwifery in North America and Europe*. New York: Routledge 139–66.

Bower, H. (2002) 'Educating the midwife', in R. Mander and V. Fleming (eds), *Failure to Progress: The Contraction of the Midwifery Profession*. London: Routledge.

Collington, V., Mallik, M., Doris, F. and Fraser, D. (2012) 'Supporting the midwifery practice-based curriculum: the role of the link lecturer'. *Nurse Education Today* 32(8): 924–9.

Dictionarist (2013) 'Scholar'. http://www.dictionarist.com/scholar. Accessed October 2013.

Hindley, C. (1997) 'From clinical credibility to academic elitism'. *British Journal of Midwifery* 5(6): 361–3.

Hunt, S.C. (1996) 'Marketing midwifery education: findings from a survey'. *Midwifery* 12(1): 31–6.

Hunt, S.C. (1998) 'Clinical credibility in midwifery education'. *British Journal of Midwifery* 6(6): 369.

Jackson, K.B. (1999) 'The role of the lecturer/practitioner in midwifery'. *British Journal of Midwifery* 7(6): 363–6.

Kenny, G., Pontin, D. and Moore, L. (2004) 'Negotiating socialisation: the journey of novice nurse academics into higher education'. *Nurse Education Today* 24(8): 629–37.

Laiho, A. (2010) 'Academisation of nursing education in the Nordic Countries'. *Higher Education* 60(6): 641–56.

MacKenzie, C. (2004) 'The politics of representation: a personal reflection on the problematic positioning of the midwifery educator'. *Studies in Continuing Education* 26(1): 117–28.

Mander, R. (1989) 'A maternity care course component and evaluation'. *Nurse Education Today* 9(4): 227–35.

Mander, R. (1992) 'The value of clinical experience to a non-clinician: combining midwifery practice with teaching'. *Midwifery* 8(4): 184–90.

Mander, R., Cheung, N.F., Wang, X., Fu, W. and Zhu, J. (2010) 'Beginning an Action Research Project to investigate the feasibility of a Midwife-Led Normal Birthing Unit in China'. *Journal of Clinical Nursing* 19(3–4): 517–26.

NMC (2010) The MINT Project NMC and University of Nottingham. London: HMSO. http://www.nmc-uk.org/Documents/Midwifery-Reports/MINT-annexe5.2.pdf. Accessed October 2013.

Thompson, D.R. and Watson, R. (2001) 'Academic nursing – what is happening to it and where is it going?' *Journal of Advanced Nursing* 36(1): 1–2.

Thompson, D.R. and Watson, R. (2006) 'Professors of nursing: what do they profess?' *Nurse Education in Practice* 6(3): 123–6.

UKCC (1994) *The Future of Professional Practice: The Council's Standards for Educational Practice Following Registration.* London: UKCC.

UKCC (2001) *Standards for Specialist Education and Practice.* London: UKCC.

Commentary

Rosemary goes straight to the hub of the matter, describing the various difficulties inherent in being a midwife academic. She writes of a phenomenon I have often encountered – the somewhat disparaging looks received if I say I am an academic. Likewise, if I encountered someone from traditional academic disciplines in the university and they ask me my subject, to respond with 'midwifery' often was met with a condescending shrug of the shoulders. Interestingly, in Switzerland where I now work, these responses do not exist. When someone working at the university is asked for her profession the answer is never academic but midwife, sociologist, accountant etc. This ensures a much more integrated approach. Rosemary also highlights another issue and that is the division of teaching, research and other functions. As she states, traditional academic disciplines tend to emphasise the research, with teaching being almost a by-product. However, when clinical skills have to be learned, as is a core requirement for midwifery, then the emphasis changes and teaching becomes more important. Rosemary has painted a picture of this dilemma and it is one which comes even more to the fore in the present climate of cost savings. It is surely essential that the midwife teaching is informed by the latest research. That is not in dispute in this chapter. What is perhaps not essential but ideal is that the most integrated midwife academic will be basing her teaching on her own research as well as that of others. Her vignette, cleverly placed at the end of the chapter, ends by showing how this view has gradually come to be accepted by a former doubting student.

8

THE MIDWIFE AS A RESEARCHER

Ans Luyben

Introduction

Once you have become a midwife, being a researcher is not the first thing that comes to your mind. Midwifery is an exciting profession. It is fascinating how a new life begins, and the individuality of a woman's experience is challenging. Newly qualified midwives therefore will primarily choose to work with pregnant women, their children and families in everyday practice. Practising midwifery not only involves scientific knowledge, but also art and caring sensitivity, in which midwives use their own personality in order to achieve positive effects in caring for mothers and their families. Whereas these magic elements are essential to care, they have been hard to capture and evaluate in studies (Enkin & Chalmers 1982). In everyday practice, however, midwives are frequently confronted with medical research, often following a reductionist, standardised approach. Many midwives experienced this kind of research in contrast to the individual approach needed for their work. Being a researcher therefore seems like a different profession.

Midwifery research addresses midwives' ways of working and aims to improve midwifery practice. If this happens, research can be as fascinating as midwifery practice itself. Well-known midwifery researchers started their first research projects with a question that arose from practice, and thus contributed to the reduction of unnecessary interventions during childbirth. Some midwives started questioning aspects of practice during their training and experienced the difference that research can make. This is how I started on my research career. Our research project on parameters for diagnosing intrauterine growth retardation (slow growth in babies) led to a reduction of the number of hormone measurements in the hospital where I worked. Motivated by this consequence, my next question again arose in practice and addressed the reduction of adverse outcomes of breech birth (Roumen & Luyben 1991). From these experiences I learnt about the importance of research evidence for practice as well as its compatibility with the art of midwifery.

Meanwhile, midwifery research has developed as a discipline. One of its greatest current strengths is the rich diversity of methods (Steen & Roberts 2011; Downe *et al.* 2012). This diversity in particular allows midwives currently to address not only the medical, but also several other aspects of midwifery practice. The objectives of this research as well as a short history of midwifery researchers are described in the next sections. Following, a picture of the role of a midwife as a researcher is presented, based on the literature, personal information from research midwives in the UK and the USA, and my own experience, as well as the experiences of three midwives involved in research in three European countries: Mechthild (Germany), Greta (the Netherlands) and Martina (Switzerland).

Why midwifery research is needed

Throughout history, midwifery knowledge had most often been orally transferred from midwife to midwife and little was documented. This way, knowledge was discovered, developed, but also lost. Only a few midwives left their knowledge in a written form, like Catharina Schrader who documented her midwifery experiences in the Netherlands during the eighteenth century as case studies (van Lieburg 1984). Until the second half of the twentieth century, however, midwifery knowledge was mainly based on authority, tradition, intuition, experience and research by other disciplines.

A call for midwifery research was raised during the 1970s and 1980s, particularly in the United States (USA) and the United Kingdom (UK). Professional questioning of the effectiveness of maternity care, as well as the involvement of consumers, indicated the need for childbirth reforms. This development coincided with the establishment of the profession of nurse-midwives in the USA and the search for recognition of their care. Meanwhile, medical professionals in the UK aimed to reduce maternal and perinatal mortality and morbidity and increase the effectiveness of interventions in maternity care through systematic evaluation, which also involved midwifery (Chalmers *et al.* 1989). As a result, the need for basing professional practice on research was emphasised.

Midwifery research therefore aims to create a body of midwifery knowledge, which underpins and improves midwifery practice, and thus maternity care, which involves:

- improving the effectiveness and quality of maternity care, which includes the provision of woman-centred care;
- expanding knowledge of the multiple aspects of a woman's childbearing process (for example, physiological, psychological, sociological) as well as the influence of maternity care on this process;
- increasing the number of options of maternity care available to women;
- increasing evidence-based practice and developing standards of maternity care;
- developing a sound basis as well as a vision for midwifery practice.

A short history of midwives as researchers

Midwifery research and the professional role of researcher only go back about three decades. Before this time, new knowledge was merely generated by researchers in other disciplines, in particular obstetricians and nurses. Reva Rubin, an American nurse for example, developed a nursing theory of becoming a mother during the 1970s (Rubin 1984). In a similar way, active management of labour is based on research from medical practitioners. Several researchers, like the team of the World Health Organization, however, stressed the need for midwives to conduct research in their own field. Following a study of maternity services in Europe during the 1970s, they stated that:

> midwives have to study the work of midwives, together with competent scientists, so that they gradually create a body of explicit midwifery knowledge and raise a group of midwifery researchers. Part of this research has to be qualitative (focusing on the everyday experience of people and using methods like interviews and observations) and will hopefully question, the contribution of lay and traditionally trained midwives to maternity care.
>
> *(WHO 1987 p. 93)*

Posts for midwifery researchers were first established in English-speaking countries, although the integration of research as a professional role and topics of research varied in these countries. In the USA, research focused on proving the effectiveness of midwifery care, including home birth, birth centres and care for vulnerable groups (Farley 2005). Some midwives documented their practical experience, like Ina May Gaskin, who systematically evaluated 82 cases of using the All-Fours Manoeuvre for reducing shoulder dystocia during labour (Bruner *et al.* 1998). In the UK, recognition of midwives as researchers particularly increased as some midwives used research to challenge issues of their everyday practice. A well-known pioneer was Jennifer Sleep, who studied the liberal performance of episiotomies (an incision into the soft tissues of the birth outlet) in a randomised controlled trial during the 1980s, while being supported by researchers from the Perinatal Epidemiology Unit in Oxford. The results showed that the number of episiotomies during labour could be reduced. Other topics addressed by midwifery researchers during the 1980s and 1990s addressed, for example, the provision of information by midwives during labour (Kirkham 1989) or pushing techniques in the second stage of labour (Thomson 1993).

In other European countries, this development happened in a later period in time, and was supported by research workshops held by midwives from the UK. In some countries, midwives succeeded in doing research as part of postgraduate study. In Sweden, Gunny Röckner (Röckner 1989) carried out a doctoral study on the frequency of episiotomies and spontaneous tears close to her retirement, although she had wanted to do research most of her professional life. Some undertook research as a member of an interdisciplinary team. In the Netherlands,

Rita Iedema-Kuiper (1996) did a doctoral study on the effectiveness of home care for women with a high-risk pregnancy in co-operation with researchers from other disciplines. Other midwives documented their experiences or carried out small research projects in midwifery practice. Gaby Sprung (1998) in Austria, studied the use of medicine during labour, and found out that a trusting relationship between midwife and woman reduced its frequency. Another important topic implemented and studied in several countries with midwives as researchers was the model of a midwife-led unit.

Current places of work of midwifery researchers

The availability of posts as midwifery researchers varies per country. Some countries, like the UK or the Netherlands, have professional or national guidelines describing the need for midwives to conduct research and mentioning this role, whereas in other countries this role is established as part of a research appointment for a Master's or doctoral study or has to be created. After doing her doctorate, Mechthild in Germany found a combined post of working as a midwife and being a research fellow under the Head of the Department of Obstetrics and Gynaecology of a German hospital. She created her new post herself and developed it into being a midwifery researcher in practice, although this is still unique in Germany.

Midwives are working as researchers in different practical settings, most often, however, in large, tertiary hospitals. Some midwives work as a research midwife, while carrying out research projects as their main occupation. These posts vary slightly depending on the kind of clinical projects involved, who is leading the project, the funding source, and whether the midwife is also working in practice or education. Some of these posts have a very temporary nature due to the time and funding of the project, which put a lot of midwives off. Other midwives are doing research as an integral part of their post, which involve practice development midwife, consultant midwife or midwifery expert, like Martina in a Swiss university hospital. Her work includes improving evidence-based practice, developing standards of midwifery care, organising courses for midwives in the hospital and carrying out research projects in co-operation with the Department of Clinical Research.

Midwives also work as researchers or midwifery experts in other health care organisations and institutions in midwifery-specific domains as well as part of an interdisciplinary team. Examples of such organisations and institutions include NHS Trusts (UK), governmental or regional health departments, institutes for health technology assessment, and the Dutch institute for research in health care (NIVEL). Greta in the Netherlands, for example, works as a midwifery expert in her position as a secretary for the Science Committee of the Royal Dutch Organisation of Midwives (KNOV). This committee aims to financially support midwives who want to do a doctoral study for becoming a researcher or develop a scientific career after doing their study. Part of her job is to ensure that research evidence will be incorporated into professional policies, and thus midwifery work.

Training

Postgraduate training should provide the midwifery researcher with the methodological and methodical competencies that she needs for carrying out research projects, which involves theory as well as practical experience. Before the establishment of research as a professional role for midwives in the UK, midwives had to identify the relevant courses themselves and most training was self-funded and had to be attended in personal time. Currently, this training is likely to be considered integral to the role and to be funded. A similar trend can be seen in other European countries.

Some agreement exists that the minimum requirement for training to prepare midwives for the role of a midwifery researcher constitutes a study at Master's level (Master's of Science or Master's of Philosophy), which include research and a research dissertation. Both Greta and Mechthild studied for a Master's degree on a part-time basis and funded it themselves. Although Martina had already started a part-time, self-funded Master's in Midwifery, for finishing the study she received study time from her employer as an integral part of the new post. The availability of the required training, however, varies by country, as in many countries a midwifery-specific Master's degree is not offered. Alternative training involves studying abroad (likely UK, USA), studying in another discipline (for example public health, nursing) or attending several relevant postgraduate courses in research (Certificate of Advanced Studies, Diploma of Advanced Studies).

Salary

As the post of the midwifery researcher is not officially established in all countries, the salary varies. The main influencing factor is the national system of wages. Additional factors that play a role in regard to the salary in different countries involves the job description, working experience as a midwife and the level of study required for the post. Most salaries are a bit higher than the salary of a midwife in practice, due to the higher requirements in regard to training. In some posts the salary of researchers increases with increased acquisition of external finances.

Everyday work

The structure of a day in the life of a midwife in the role of a researcher depends on her job description. A midwife doing research as an integral part of a post (for example practice development midwife) will have a different structure of a working day than a midwifery researcher who is working on a project full time. This researcher might have her own project, but also work as a member of a larger team. She usually has her own project plan to follow and go through in an autonomous, but sometimes also solitary way. Others, like Greta in the Netherlands, participate in several other projects, while working together with obstetricians, neonatologists, epidemiologists and midwives.

A normal day might be working from nine to five, but depending on the project plan and the stage of the project, it might also involve working till late or even being on call. Such a day, for example while working on a clinical trial in the postnatal ward, might involve discussing the research with women, seeing whether there are any new research participants, collecting clinical samples and data, documenting these data, reading related research papers and discussing the study with colleagues or students. Whereas a clinical trial might involve collecting clinical samples and data in the hospital, a qualitative study could involve interviewing women at home. A lot of time in research is also involved in analysing data, documenting the study and writing up the results. For some research midwives their working day might also involve professional development related to the project and/or their post, as well as acquisition of new projects with external funding. Although improvement of care for mothers and babies is high on the agenda on the United Nations (Millenium Development Goals 4 and 5), finding financial support for maternity care projects in Europe is not easy.

Depending on the position of the midwifery researcher in the hospital, sometimes other clinical staff activities (meetings, audits, presentations) are integrated in the working day. As a midwifery expert, Martina in Switzerland has a variety of clinical roles integrated in her job. Therefore her everyday activities involve counselling colleagues, evaluating case studies of midwifery care, developing, implementing and evaluating practice programmes and standards, and of course, research.

Projects

The post of a research midwife in practice is often related to an institution's objectives to initiate research projects in midwifery and obstetrics/gynaecology, or an existing project (or part of a project) that needs to be carried out by a midwifery researcher. Mechthild, for example, pursued her doctoral project on influential factors on the birth process, such as rupture of membranes or pain relief, in her new job, and she managed to involve a few other regional hospitals. Mechtild's post was financed by the hospital but also involved the acquisition of external funding.

Many small projects are (and have been) carried out by midwives doing research as an integral part of their posts. The questions for these projects arise directly from midwifery practice and directly feed back to it. For these smaller projects, financing is often not a particular issue, and midwives are working on them as part of their job. Some projects initiated in practice might, however, grow bigger, and such is the research role of the midwife. A good example for such a project has been the implementation of a midwife-led unit. Turnbull et al. (1996) evaluated the outcomes of midwife-led care compared with traditional care during labour for low-risk women in a Scottish hospital. The study concluded that this model of care was clinically effective, while women in the midwife-led unit had the same or lower rates of interventions and were more satisfied than women with traditional care. Following this study, several midwife-led units were implemented in other

European countries (Austria, Switzerland and Germany) (Schuster 1998; Cignacco *et al.* 2004; Bauer & zu Sayn-Wittgenstein 2006). As this new model of care was a political issue in these countries, the implementation of the units had to be accompanied by research, and this thus raised the need for research midwives.

The projects mentioned above are only a few examples of research carried out by midwives in practice. A complete overview of international midwifery research is hard to create, due to the fact that midwives are not always the lead researcher, and they also participate in research projects of medical practitioners and collect sample (such as blood or amniotic fluid) data during their work in the birthing room. Following the development and establishment of the professional role of the midwife in research, however, the Midwifery Research Database was initiated in the UK. The publication MIRIAD (Simms *et al.* 1994), based on the data collected in this database, provides an overview of midwifery research projects carried out in the UK during the last decades, and is a good example for documentation of professional research by midwives.

Networking and co-operation

Networks are essential for doing midwifery research for a variety of reasons. Primarily, they are necessary for having the direct support for doing one's own research, which involves having access to both experts for counselling as well as statistical and computer support. In some countries, this support network is available in the institutions where research takes place, whereas in other countries researchers have to create it themselves, often related with extra costs. Without such a supporting network, however, it is almost impossible to carry out a research project.

A second reason for needing a network is the opportunity to discuss the study and exchange knowledge in regard to the research topic, as well as the dissemination of the results of the study.

Being located in a university hospital, Martina and Mechthild work with midwifery, medical and research colleagues, and have the opportunity for presentation of their study, discussion and exchange. Greta is part of a midwifery research network, and collaborates with several national research groups.

Conferences also provide an adequate platform for dissemination of a study, and in particular for getting to know, and discussing with, other researchers who are addressing a similar topic. Another valuable international platform to present one's study, discuss it with midwifery colleagues and get expert opinions, is the Midwifery Research List (http://www.jiscmail.ac.uk). Some countries have created their own platform for midwifery research. For example, the midwifery schools in the Netherlands created a national web-based platform. Kennispoort Verloskunde (http//:www.kennispoort-verloskunde.nl) not only provides an overview of midwifery research, but also studies in maternity care carried out by researchers from other disciplines.

Careers

As the role of the midwife as a researcher is a rather new phenomenon, little is known about career possibilities. The careers of the earliest midwifery researchers in the UK were related to the new professional orientation of midwifery. Having their research published in international peer-reviewed professional journals, such as *Birth*, *Midwifery* and the *Journal of Midwifery and Women's Health*, has been an important means for getting them known. Some found a post within research units affiliated with universities or large health care institutions, such as the Perinatal Epidemiology Unit in Oxford. Others took up a post in a university as a lecturer, researcher or head of a midwifery school or department of health sciences. Best known are the research midwives who become professors, either through the need for professors in midwifery as a result of moving into higher education or a step-wise academic career in research and education.

Other possible careers for research midwives involve management in a hospital, such as head of a department, or manager or expert positions in health care institutions or organisations, for example, the World Health Organization. Being such a new role, new jobs might develop which cannot be imagined at this moment, or as one of the research midwives in this chapter wrote in regard to her career, 'the future will tell.'

Acknowledgements

Many thanks to Mechthild Gross, Martina Gisin, Helen Spiby and Greta Rijninks-van Driel for sharing their experiences.

References

Bauer, N. and Sayn-Wittgenstein, F. zu (2006) 'Hebammenkreißsaal: Besonderheiten eines randomisiert, kontrollierten Studiendesigns'. *Die Hebamme* 19(2): 107–9.

Bruner, J.P., Drummond, S., Meenan, A.I., and Gaskin, I.M. (1998) 'The all-fours manoeuvre for reducing shoulder dystocia during labour'. *Journal of Reproductive Medicine* 43: 433–9.

Chalmers, I., Enkin, M. and Keirse, M.J.N.C. (1989) *Effective Care in Pregnancy and Childbirth.* Oxford: Oxford University Press.

Cignacco, E., Büchi, S. and Oggier, W. (2004) 'Hebammengeleitete Geburtshilfe in einem Schweizer Spital'. *Pflege* 17(5): 253–61.

Downe, S., Thomson, G. and Dykes, F. (2012) *Qualitative Research in Midwifery and Childbirth. Phenomenological Approaches.* London: Routledge.

Enkin, M. and Chalmers, I. (1982) 'Effectiveness and satisfaction in antenatal care', in M. Enkin and I. Chalmers (eds), *Effectiveness and Satisfaction in Antenatal Care.* London: Heinemann Medical Ltd, pp. 266–90.

Farley, C.L. (2005) 'Midwifery's research heritage: a Delphi survey of midwife scholars'. *Journal of Midwifery and Women's Health* 50(2): 122–28.

Iedema-Kuiper, H.R. (1996) 'Geïntegreerde thuiszorg bij risico-zwangeren' ['Domiciliary risk in high risk pregnancies'], Doctoral thesis, Utrecht: Universiteit Utrecht.

Kirkham, M.J. (1989) 'Midwives and information-giving during labour', in S. Robinson and A.M. Thomson (eds), *Midwives, Research and Childbirth.* London: Chapman and Hall, Vol. 1, pp. 117–38.

van Lieburg, M.J. (1984) *C.G. Schrader's Memoryboeck van de vrouwens*, Amsterdam: Rodopi.

Röckner, G. (1989) 'Episiotomy and perineal trauma during childbirth'. *Journal of Advanced Nursing* 14: 264–68.

Roumen, F.J.M.E. and Luyben, A.G. (1991) 'Safety of the term vaginal breech delivery'. *European Journal of Obstetrics & Gynaecology and Reproductive Biology* 40(3): 171–7.

Rubin, R. (1984) *Maternal identity and the maternal experience*, New York: Springer Publishing Company.

Schuster, U. (1998) 'Hebammengeburtshilfe- Ein Projekt an der Universittsklinik Wien'. *Oesterreichische Hebammenzeitung* 5: 152–3.

Simms, C., McHaffie, H., Renfrew, M. and Ashurst, H. (1994) *The Midwifery Research Database. MIRIAD. A sourcebook of information about research in midwifery*, Hale: Book for Midwives.

Sprung, G. (1998) 'Medikamentengabe während der Geburt. Ein Hebammenforschungsprojekt am KH Korneuburg'. *Oesterreichische Hebammenzeitung* 6: 167–8.

Steen. M. and Roberts, T. (2011) *The Handbook of Midwifery Research*. Chichester: Wiley-Blackwell.

Thomson, A.M. (1993) 'Pushing techniques in the second stage of labour'. *Journal of Advanced Nursing*, 18: 171–7.

Turnbull, D., Holmes, A., Shields, N., Cheyne, H., Twaddle, S., Harper Gilmour, W. *et al.* (1996) 'Randomised, controlled trial of efficacy of midwife-managed care'. *Lancet* 348(9022): 213–8.

World Health Organization (WHO) (1987) *Wenn ein Kind unterwegs ist . . . Bericht über eine Studie*, Oeffentliches Gesundheitswesen in Europa 26, World Health Organization Regional Office for Europe: Copenhagen.

Commentary

Ans achieves the remarkable feat of making sense of a complicated and rapidly changing aspect of midwifery. While, for many people, the picture of research work comprises attending conferences in exotic destinations, the reality is likely to be very different. As Ans explains, conferences matter for a number of reasons, but they are only a small part of what research is about. The researcher is certainly likely to enjoy the elation of a well-received conference presentation or the publication of a paper in a peer-reviewed journal. The work that is necessary to achieve that elation may be considerably less attractive, possibly featuring travelling, working late or rescheduling appointments with participants who find difficulty meeting the researcher. The highs and lows of research will also involve submitting carefully prepared grant applications. Increasingly, the researcher will find that their proposal has been rejected, not because it is faulty in any way, but simply because of the huge volume of marginally better applications. Similarly, the researcher must submit their proposal for management and ethical approval, to teams whose understanding of research may appear to be less than complete. Although research ethics committees have endeavoured to make their functioning more effective, there still appears to be some way to go (Schrag 2011).

Reference

Schrag, Z.M. (2011) 'The case against ethics review in the social sciences'. *Research Ethics* 7(4): 120–31. http://rea.sagepub.com/content/7/4/120.full.pdf+html

9

THE GLOBAL MIDWIFE

Valerie Fleming

As a child, one of the highlights of a summer holiday to visit grandparents in the south west of Scotland was to be taken to the local airport during the busy holiday weekend. Where I lived I had occasionally been shown a trail of white cloud and told it came from a plane. From the observation area my brother and I scanned the skies to see what a plane really looked like. I fantasised about where they were coming from and what sort of people would go on them. Certainly no one in my circle would ever have such opportunities! Several years later, now living in south west Scotland I worked as a bus conductress to supplement my student income. To my delight I was put on the route that went past the airport. Approximately once per hour we stopped right in front of the terminal building and, at some point during that year, I vowed I would get on a plane. That opportunity arose just after I had completed my midwifery training, whereupon I embarked on a rail tour round Europe for my holidays. The only possible way I could cram it all in and be back in time for night duty was to fly from London to Aberdeen. Despite that flight living up to all my expectations, I little believed that 6 months later I would be embarking on a global career, which has now spanned several decades and every continent. As I write this chapter, I am sitting at my desk in Switzerland, where I am now based.

As with all the other career paths outlined in this book, becoming a 'global midwife' is a combination of a desire to do the job, achieving the right qualifications, experience and expertise and working to achieve the goals. This is coupled with being in the right place at the right time but also being aware of the opportunities or even creating these. It is my intention to outline in this chapter the possibilities that exist for midwives to take a global role and how they may go about achieving this. I intend to use my own experiences and those of other midwives, some of whom I encounter in a variety of places, as illustrations.

Becoming a midwife

From 1996 until 2005 a common definition of the midwife was agreed upon by the major bodies of the World Health Organization (WHO), International Confederation of Midwives (ICM) and International Federation of Obstetricians and Gynaecologists (FIGO) (WHO/ICM/FIGO 2005). This paved the way for all member states of the various bodies to offer a common base for midwifery education and a framework for practice. However, the reality is that there are numerous different programmes leading to qualification as a midwife. For example, in the UK one becomes a midwife only in a university, either through a 3-year programme or, for those who have previously qualified as nurses, a programme of 18 months. This is in complete contrast to Germany, where there is very little university education for midwives and the 3-year programme is undertaken in a vocational secondary school. Elsewhere in Europe countries such as Switzerland and Ireland offer 4-year direct entry programmes at universities.

Further afield, in countries such as India and South Africa, students complete programmes of 4 academic years at university to become nurse–midwives and, in Jordan, the programme consists of 1 year in a military hospital on completion of a nursing programme. Already difficulties can be seen in the recognition of qualifications. How can a midwife with a 6-month obstetric placement as part of a nursing programme possibly be equivalent to one with a 3- to 4-year bachelor's degree focused entirely on midwifery? It is therefore absolutely vital, for anyone entering midwifery with a view to travelling, that they ensure that their qualification will be recognised in the country in which they want to work. This hit home to me when I had almost completed my nursing programme (the only way to enter midwifery in the 1970s) and the senior tutor came into our class saying that a new Common Market (as the European Union (EU) was then) regulation had been passed stating that nurses in one EU country could now work in any other provided that they had done geriatrics. As this was not part of our curriculum, she wanted to know if any of us were interested in an elective placement there. While I was not aware of it at the time, that was Directive 77/453/EEC (EEC 1977) and a similar one was passed for midwifery 3 years later – 80/154/EEC (EEC 1980a). Midwifery went even further with another directive specifying minimum standards (EEC 1980b).

Each of these regulations has been amended on several occasions, the latest being 2005/36/EC (EU 2005), at which time all health professions were brought together under the one regulation. The midwifery specifications, however, still incorporate the minimum standards. Indeed, if any nurse thinking of becoming a midwife through a programme in the UK with the purpose of working in mainland Europe is reading this chapter, she would be advised to read this directive, as the UK qualification falls short of the minimum requirements and a period of consolidation is required. At present the directive is undergoing a major review with entry requirements to all the health professional education likely to be changed to university standard.

The 1980 directive marked the beginning of automatic recognition of midwifery education in one EU country by another. A midwife qualifying in Germany, for example, can work in France and one qualifying in Bulgaria in the UK. This is dependent upon language skills, but these may not always be appropriately tested and I have recently heard of examples of midwives imported from one country to another who cannot communicate with the women. On another recent occasion I met a newly qualified midwife from an EU country who, despite the directive, had never seen a birth during her 4 years of university education. Recognising her education to be defective, she had apprenticed herself to an experienced midwife but others in her class had not taken this option. The potential for dangerous practice is therefore high.

Although in 1977 I did not consciously harbour notions of working in another European country, I chose to do the geriatric placement, thereby gaining a really valuable experience in basic nursing. Now, in the UK, things are very different. Not only are we governed by the EU regulations that inform those of the Nursing and Midwifery Council (NMC), but since our education takes place in universities, we also have to consider the Declaration of Bologna (1999). In this, ministers of 29 countries agreed to comparable university degrees, thus creating opportunities for university-educated midwives to advance their education in other signatory countries (numbering 47 as from 2011). The countries that are signatories to this declaration vastly outnumber those of the EU. This carries the danger that while academic qualifications must be recognised in the signatory countries, potentially professional qualifications are not. For the midwife wanting to work in one of the countries this affects, this may well mean much negotiation.

Potential for midwives early in their careers

Although the midwifery directive was passed just after I had completed my education, it was never alluded to either during or after I had completed the programme. One thing that was certain, however, after my first experience of European travel and flying, was that I wanted to travel. A few opportunities presented themselves through advertisements in professional journals, but all of them required considerably more experience than I had. Other options were with voluntary groups, such as Voluntary Service Overseas (VSO), but many of these were, and still are, for 2-year periods, often in uncomfortable settings. At that stage, I was not convinced it was for me, but there are many midwives whom I have subsequently met who have found such experiences immensely valuable and have built their entire careers working in similar organisations.

My own plans were made together with an Australian midwife with whom I shared a flat. We planned an ambitious trip through western Asia to India and south east Asia, ending up at my friend's home. Thereafter, I would fly back and fulfil my ambition to become a ward sister. However, it very quickly became evident that money was an obstacle and, to do this dream trip, I would have to work for an agency on my days off and find employment in Australia before returning. At that time Australia was only issuing 1-year visas with no guarantee of renewal, so I opted instead for New Zealand, which wanted midwives (but not nurses) and was prepared to offer me permanent residence. While I have glossed over this issue in one sentence, it is important to say that, for anyone in the same position now, this did not happen easily. In some ways, it may be easier now, since the advent of the internet, but it is still time-consuming and even more bureaucratic. Negotiations must be made with prospective employers, consulates and midwifery regulatory bodies. Clearly, where regulatory bodies exist, potential global midwives must check with them that their qualifications will be recognised or, if not, if the requirements are acceptable. Often requirements involve a period of continuing education for which a fee is charged and during which the midwife cannot practise. In turn, this may make immigration difficult, as a job offer will not be made until the qualification is obtained. While this may appear to be a vicious circle, it is usually possible through sharing all the correspondence with each of the parties concerned to reach a compromise. However, the fundamental driver will always be the labour market at the time, and such was the case in 1980 when my friend and I finally made some of our epic journey though Asia.

Wars and invasions meant that our plans to travel through western Asia had to be abandoned and, instead, we flew to India to begin a 3-month exploration of the subcontinent. I was affected greatly by the poverty, masses of people and the bureaucracy there and, after 2 weeks, desperately wanted to escape. However, I persisted and eventually in my travels reached Tiruneveli in Tamil Nadu, where I had been in contact already with a doctor known to one of my colleagues in Aberdeen. When we met her she was delighted that two midwives had come to see her and took us to the hospital where she worked. On the door were the mortality statistics for the month and, to someone who had only ever seen one maternal death, they were frightening, while to this doctor they were a vast improvement. She felt that they could be much better if there were sufficient midwives to work there. Naturally we volunteered and suddenly we were there, earning no money but a wealth of experience. We were not registered with the Indian Nursing Council, but such was the need that this was irrelevant to the local authorities. The labour market had dictated what was required and we were in the right place.

The same could be said for my next placement on the Thai-Kampuchean border. Civil war had broken out in Cambodia and refugees were flooding over the border into Thailand in the hope of escaping persecution. Infectious diseases such as cholera and typhoid were endemic and, as I was nearby and had been vaccinated, I felt I could be of some use. The International Red Cross was delighted to see me and, once more, I felt able to be of use while building up my own experience.

It was therefore as a much more experienced midwife than I had anticipated that I finally arrived in New Zealand, where I mixed with a large group of global midwives, most of whom had come on 1-year working visas. I was delighted to have my permanent residency, however, as I stayed in New Zealand for 16 years, pursuing a more recognisable career working as a midwife in various settings. Two exemplars stand out, however, that have relevance for the aspiring global midwife of today. Four years after I had arrived in New Zealand, I decided on a trip back to the UK to visit family. At that point I discovered that permanent residence was only permanent as long as I stayed in the country. The authorities no longer had any need of midwives, so residence would not be renewed. My solution was to apply for (and gain) citizenship. Dual nationality in my career today is extremely useful!

The second example was my own drive to improve my education. New Zealand offered opportunities that the UK did not at that time and I pursued first an Advanced Diploma of Midwifery and thereafter a bachelor's degree by distance learning. With the Declaration of Bologna and other systems in place for recognition of prior learning in many countries, for midwives to gain a bachelor's degree is relatively straightforward and may involve as little as one semester's full-time study. However, in the 1980s it involved 4 years of full-time equivalent study to gain those two qualifications. What they did was make me want to learn more and, before leaving New Zealand, I had gained my PhD, had a good career record, had learned a lot about international health, in particular women's health, and had the confidence to apply for a position back in Scotland in what the advert called a 'World Health Organisation Collaborating Centre'. I was successful in attaining that position and for 15 years worked as an academic midwife while simultaneously pursuing an international career.

Global opportunities

There are perhaps more opportunities for midwives to pursue international careers now than ever before. Prevailing health problems that continue to face many regions include the increasing gap between the health of the rich and poor and unacceptable mortality/morbidity statistics. In addition, there is a resurgence of many infectious diseases, for example tuberculosis, meningitis and hepatitis, as well as sexually transmissible diseases, such as HIV/AIDS, and their associated problems. Many countries and communities are faced with women with lifestyle-related problems, such as unhealthy diets, too little exercise, smoking and alcohol and substance misuse. Increasing numbers of some populations suffer from stress, mental ill health and other chronic diseases, while others face the effects of poverty and unemployment (Fleming and Holmes 2005). The opportunities are thus plentiful for both midwives with little experience and those with many years of working at senior levels. Both have valuable contributions to make and positions can be short or long term, paid or voluntary. For the remainder of this chapter I intend to outline some of these possibilities.

Crisis situations

In the various news media, we are faced almost daily with stories of natural disasters and civil wars. While the plea is often for money or equipment, there is always a need for human resources and midwives are particularly valuable, as many populations outside the western world include young women who often have been trafficked and/or sexually abused. Women, too, are frequently considered of lesser importance than men or children and their health needs do not receive priority assistance locally in times of crisis. The voluntary aid organisations are among those that do their best to fill these gaps. Some of these are faith-based, while others are secular in their orientation; midwives aspiring to work with such organisations need to recognise this to ensure that their own beliefs do not clash with those of the organisation with which they propose to work. As I found to my cost in a large international organisation, these beliefs are not always made clear until policies are drilled down and their cores reached.

Any midwife planning to work in crisis situations needs to have not only the professional and technical skills to carry out the job, but also needs to be strongly aware of local cultural beliefs and values in order to embrace these or, at the very least, not cause offence with certain practices. Perhaps one of the strongest examples of this is the practice of female genital mutilation (FGM), which takes place in many parts of Africa and elsewhere. Girls, either shortly after birth or any time until they reach puberty, have their external genitalia excised to varying degrees, the stated aim being to keep them celibate in preparation for marriage. When sexual intercourse does take place it is usually extremely painful for the woman and often leads to chronic urinary and genital infections. When the woman with a more radical form of FGM gives birth, it is necessary to reverse this mutilation in order for the baby to be born safely. After the birth, the woman or her husband frequently requests that she is returned to her pre-birth state. While most western countries have outlawed such a practice, it remains the norm for many women in some of the countries in which midwives will work; increasingly in Europe it is being experienced amongst refugees from sub-Saharan Africa. Midwives going to work in times of crisis in such areas need to be aware of this, and other similar practices, and deal only with the crisis, while remembering that many international organisations are working on a long-term basis together with concerned local groups and individuals in an attempt to change such practices.

Midwives working in crisis situations are generally responding to some specific emergency and will find themselves working and living in horrific conditions. It is essential to be aware of this before agreeing to embark upon such work as, once in the affected area, there is generally little chance of opting out and returning home without causing a lot of difficulties and expense to all concerned. However, the rewards of such work are substantial, not only through the immediate help that can be given to women and their families, but also by working in the multidisciplinary teams that are the norm at such times. The benefits of working in such teams include the sharing of knowledge and experience, as well as the making of lasting friendships and finding out about where the next job opportunity might be.

Indeed, midwives, and of course others, choosing to work in crisis situations would not be doing their jobs properly if their postings were long term. To work in a crisis situation means to go in as part of a rescue effort and deliver the appropriate package. As mentioned above, there are many crisis situations in the world, and it is often the same group of people who move from one to the next, thereby building up a body of experience and expertise that is immediately transferable.

Although I have talked about the voluntary aid organisations in this section, it does not always mean that a midwife's work in crisis situations is unpaid. Indeed, in some instances a highly attractive salary may be offered. As with any other position, it is vital to ensure well in advance what the terms and conditions of employment are to facilitate informed choice.

Reconstruction

While responding to crisis situations is something that happens rapidly, reconstruction usually comes about following much negotiation with governments and large organisations, which are often, although not exclusively, agencies of the United Nations (UN), such as the WHO or UNICEF. Other major stakeholders in reconstruction work are frequently international banks, such as the World or Asian Development Banks, while yet others are individual governments of wealthier countries or foundations launched by philanthropists, such as the Aga Khan Foundation or the Bill and Melinda Gates Foundation, while several faith-based organisations contribute. To the outsider, reconstruction work may often appear to be fragmented and lacking in coordination, resulting in duplication of effort. Indeed, this was an issue raised frequently by respondents worldwide to the UK's Department for International Development research consultation (DFID 2008).

Often, reconstruction work lasts for several years and is based on promoting public health or, more recently and more specifically, achieving the Millennium Development Goals (UN 2000). Stakeholders committed themselves to achieving these eight goals by 2015 and many countries in the world, most noticeably in the Far East, have made enormous strides and expect to achieve all the goals on target. For other countries, the outlook is not so positive and, at the midterm evaluation, several countries advised that at least one (and in some cases several) more of the goals would not be achievable by 2015 unless huge amounts of international aid were given. Three of the goals are directly concerned with women's health: these being numbers 3 to 5:

3   promote gender equality and empower women;
4   reduce child mortality;
5   improve maternal health.

Sadly, out of the eight goals, that which is least likely to be achieved is goal number 5. In most cases, this is due to a lack of skilled birth attendants who can provide adequate antenatal care, so midwives can make a vast difference by working for both large and small organisations to help improve the dreadful birth statistics that still dominate some parts of the world. The WHO's (2012) report states that maternal mortality has been reduced only by 3.1 per cent annually since 1990. This is only half as much as required to achieve MDG 5. For example, the extremes of maternal mortality ratios (WHO 2012) stand at 1,100/100,000 in Chad, compared with 2/100,000 Estonia. In developing countries generally, the figures are 450/100,000 in comparison with 9/100,000 in developed countries. In Europe we cannot afford to be complacent as, while the Estonian statistics are exemplary, they show an unusually high drop from previous years and in the Commonwealth of Independent States (CIS, former Soviet Union countries) the maternal mortality rate is still over 50/100,000.

Working with statistics such as these can be an intimidating task and midwives need to choose carefully the type of work to which they feel the most suited. In some of the smaller organisations, for example, a midwife might find herself the only 'international' at a remote field station with very little equipment. While this may be very daunting and lonely, it provides an opportunity for midwives to exercise all their clinical skills, often in very difficult situations. Many women or their families will not seek professional assistance until they have exhausted all the other possibilities and, if they do approach the foreign midwife, it is often with suspicion. Care therefore needs to be taken by midwives when posted to remote field stations to ensure that they become fully conversant with local beliefs and practices and do not immediately set out to contradict these. As shown earlier in this chapter, FGM is commonplace in parts of Africa with latest UN statistics (2007) showing that 97.5 per cent of women are subjected to some degree of this practice.

The midwife who is working in a long-term capacity is ideally placed to begin re-education of women in this situation, working slowly with local people of influence to build up trust and acceptance and by being willing to listen and in turn learn from local culture. Rather than being entirely on their own, however, midwives working for small organisations may often find themselves lodging with other professionals (often engineers) working for the same or other organisations. This makes them part of a small community, not only sharing accommodation but also aspirations and ideals. A close-knit community such as this is almost like a family, accompanied by its own highs and lows.

Finding such positions often comes by word of mouth and, as mentioned earlier; frequently the same group of people may be seen moving from project to project. That can only happen once a midwife has become established and is known to be capable of producing good results. The reverse may happen, where a midwife who has not been successful is unable to find other similar employment. To enter such positions for the first time often means a good deal of determination and patience, as vacancies are frequently not advertised.

If midwives simply want the experience of working for such organisations and do not mind which, they have more scope. They still need to trawl through many websites and write to numerous people. If they feel more restricted, for example in terms of working with religious organisations or those with a particular philosophy, they will have less searching to do but less potential. Working for some of the larger organisations, such as the UN's various agencies, offers different possibilities. Applications are made via a standard competitive process. Qualifications such as master's degrees are often sought. However, such agencies may offer the possibility of internships during master's degrees to raise awareness of the agencies and the type of work that they offer. These are generally unpaid positions, but the intern will be attached to a specific programme and may get the chance to visit the areas where the project is taking place. For example, in 2007, when I was working with the WHO on a project, a regional meeting was held in Zambia. All the interns working for the project were included in that meeting, thereby gaining first-hand experience of working at a strategic level within this large organisation.

Midwives may be employed by these agencies for specific projects that are likely to be based in their headquarters or in the various regional offices. Country offices nearly always employ local people, though 'internationals' may be seconded for varying periods of time. The specific project for which a midwife will be employed will reflect not only skills as a midwife but the education and experience she has subsequently received. For example, an initiative known as 'Making Pregnancy Safer' is supported by several agencies and midwives employed on that project may be employees of any of the organisations involved but are most likely to be required to be an expert in education, international health or in leading teams of people. Working for such large organisations, particularly at the level of individual projects, nearly always involves temporary contracts but, as with the smaller organisations, there are generally opportunities to move from project to project depending on the strength of experience, expertise and track record.

Another way in which midwives can become involved with the work of large organisations is not to work for them but to work with them. Most of my own recent experience has been in this area, so I intend to finish this chapter in the way in which I started it; that is, by outlining some of the recent projects I have run in recent years and showing how I managed to win the tenders for these projects and carry them out.

As indicated earlier in the chapter, I chose to join a university department that was a WHO Collaborating Centre (WHOCC). I had little real sense of what this meant, but quickly made it my business to find out. I made sure that the Centre's director was aware of work I had done and where I felt I could be useful. I was privileged to be invited to the biennial meeting of the Global Network of Collaborating Centres, where I was able to see the group in action and establish contacts with those people who shared my interests in women's health. During this time, I was continuing to develop my profile as an academic and improve my foreign language skills. In turn, this led me to other international meetings, where I continued to build up a network of contacts, thereby securing a secondment to a German university for a semester as a visiting professor. In turn, this led to more contacts, some of whom subsequently worked with me on other funded projects.

Another important contact was a nurse from Jordan who was Dean of an academic faculty and was keen to establish academic midwifery in her country. Much email discussion followed and, some 2 years later, we were awarded a grant from the British Council for 4 years to develop a programme, the graduates of which later studied for doctoral degrees in the UK and elsewhere. Through management of the programme, I was invited in 2007 to run a pre-doctoral programme for a group of Palestinian nurses and midwives with master's degrees. This programme was jointly sponsored by the WHO, an Israeli university, an external agency and my employing institution.

As a direct result of our WHOCC status, I (by this stage the Centre's deputy director) was invited to tender along with all the other WHOCCs in Europe to do a scoping study on reconstructing midwifery and nursing education in post-war Kosovo. We won this tender and, after carrying out the work, were invited to implement it. This was a much harder task, but provided experience for many of my colleagues and those from other institutions who had not previously had such opportunities. All of them spent from 1 to 6 months in Kosovo working with locals, while I commuted, spending 1 week per month there. It was a proud moment when, after 3 difficult years, our first graduates received their degrees.

I have carried out a number of other consultancies for WHO and other organisations, during which I have come across other consultants. Some of these are freelance and others employees. In both the education and clinical fields, I believe that freelance consultants have a career lifespan of approximately 2 years (though others would dispute this), as ideas are changing so rapidly that knowledge quickly becomes outdated. Midwives need to decide how they are going to stay in touch with these changes if they are going to freelance long term. Additionally, midwives spending any length of time in countries other than their own need to decide whether they are going to be part of the international community, or whether to spend more time with locals. During my time in Kosovo, as with other projects, I made many friends, mostly from among the Kosovars, but there was also a thriving British community that had activities of its own as well as its own favourite haunts for nightlife!

Conclusion

In this chapter, I have shown many of my own experiences in order to illustrate the rich tapestry of opportunities available to midwives seeking to become global in their own approach to their work. Both the projects I have mentioned above and the many other consultancies I have run for various stakeholders have involved an incredible amount of hard work; indeed shift work did not end when I moved into academic life! There are also many disappointments, as much work gets invested in preparing research proposals or tenders for funding only to be rejected by those with the money. At times, when waiting in an uncomfortable airport for 6 hours in the middle of the night, I question myself. However, it is extremely rewarding work and begets ever more work.

References

Declaration of Bologna (1999) *Joint Declaration of European Ministers of Education*, 19 June.

Department for International Development (DFID) (2008) *Research Strategy 2008–13*. London: Crown Copyright.

European Economic Community (EEC) (1977) *Directive Concerning Mutual Recognition of Nursing Qualifications*, Directive 77/453/EEC. Brussels: EEC.

European Economic Community (EEC) (1980a) *Directive Concerning Mutual Recognition of Midwifery Qualifications*, Directive 80/154/EEC. Brussels: EEC.

European Economic Community (EEC) (1980b) *Directive Defining Minimum Standards in Midwifery Education*, Directive 80/155/EEC. Brussels: EEC.

European Union (EU) (2005) *Directive Concerning Mutual Recognition of Health Service Professionals' Education*, Directive 2005/36/EC. Brussels: EU.

Fleming, V. and Holmes, A. (2005) *Basic Nursing and Midwifery Education in Europe*. Copenhagen: WHO.

United Nations (UN) (2000) *Millennium Development Goals*. Geneva: UN.

World Health Organization (WHO) (2012) *World Health Statistics 2012*. Online. Available at: http://www.who.int/gho/publications/world_health_statistics/EN_WHS2012_Full.pdf. Accessed 11 January 2013.

World Health Organization/International Confederation of Midwives/International Federation of Gynecology and Obstetrics (WHO/ICM/FIGO) (2005) *Definition of the Midwife*. Geneva: WHO.

Commentary

Valerie's account paints a vivid picture of a midwifery role that is very different from the one we usually envisage. Her writing creates an impression of a 'can do' approach, for which we lesser mortals just stand in awe. Her penultimate sentence, though, shows us that such a jet-setting lifestyle may be something other than just high flying! As well as the good news about all of the benefits, Valerie provides priceless insights into the reality of working in less than familiar settings. Thus the pitfalls begin to emerge. Her harrowing account of the widespread practice of 'female genital mutilation' (FGM) brings home the sensitivity of practising in an unfamiliar location. The midwife working in the UK is likely occasionally to attend a woman who has been subjected to this form of abuse. The UK midwife's position is in some ways very different from that of the midwife, described by Valerie, who is endeavouring to continue to provide care in a developing country.

The sensitivity of the situations in which the global midwife practises will only serve to make that practice even more challenging. A high level of political skills, in the sense of the dictionary definition of 'astutely contriving' is necessary as well as well-honed interpersonal skills. It may be that Politics with a capital 'P' will also feature in other aspects of the global midwife's work (Mander & Murphy-Lawless 2013). This possibility may be gleaned from Valerie's mention of some of the countries to which she travels and the international organisations with whom she works.

Thus, political skills and supreme sensitivity are the qualifications needed for the global midwife. Such skills and sensitivity are essential to allow effective decisions to be made in 'prickly' situations. This applies particularly to situations involving cultural practices that we might ordinarily find abhorrent, or when working with countries or agencies whose regimes are antithetical to our own principles. Thus, it is apparent that global midwives, perhaps like their more earth-bound co-professionals, need to have a very clear vision of their personal objectives. This vision will help these midwives to address the priorities that are important to them and the women and families with whom they work. Identifying such priorities will help them to address the crucial needs of the women and their babies, while other levels and agencies focus on the less manageable factors.

Reference

Mander, R. and Murphy-Lawless, J. (2013) *The Politics of Maternity*. London: Routledge.

10

THE INDEPENDENT AND NON-NHS MIDWIFE

Nessa McHugh

VIGNETTE 1

7am: I am on my way to visit Beth; her partner Andy, has phoned to say that Beth's labour has built up and she would now like me to visit. Having spoken to Beth I think she is right. I have already contacted Allison, my midwifery partner, to let her know what is happening so that she can plan her day and get her children off to school.

7.40am: I arrive at Beth's house; the last couple of miles are up a farm track and as I get out of the car I can see right across the valley – it is a beautiful morning. When I go in to see Beth, the lights are low and there is soft music playing in the background. Beth looks like she is labouring well and Andy is massaging her, whispering encouragement as another contraction washes over her. Quickly and quietly I bring my birth kit into the house and get everything I need organised, being careful not to disturb Beth with my activity.

I contact Allison again to let her know that I think Beth appears to be in good labour.

8.00am: Beth is in the pool and I have written down my observations and plan of care. As labour intensifies Andy and Beth's sister, Sarah, are with Beth supporting her through each contraction. I stay in the background, observing and waiting until I am needed.

8.15am: Beth starts the deep groaning of all women who are getting ready to give birth. There is a subtle shift in the atmosphere, Beth is now holding on to her sister as she breathes through the contractions. Allison silently appears in the room. We make eye contact but say nothing.

8.20am: Beth leans forward in the pool and I look into the eyes of her baby as her head emerges into the water. I can hear Andy telling Beth he can see the baby. At the next contraction, Beth gives a small grunt and her baby slithers out and she reaches down to greet her new daughter, Ruby.

8.30am: As Ruby nuzzles Beth, the placenta separates and is caught in a nearby bowl.

11am: Beth is lying on her bed with Ruby. Jamie her little boy has arrived with Grandma and is sat on the bed inspecting his new sister.

Allison and I retreat to the kitchen to finish writing up our notes and to ensure that the family enjoy some privacy together.

It is a beautiful day to be born.

Introduction

This chapter is an account of my experience of practising as an independent midwife. My practice enabled me to choose to carry a small caseload of women and provide backup for other midwives whilst also continuing to work as a midwifery lecturer. The above vignette provides a snapshot of the intimacy of midwifery practice, where the midwife has had the time to get to know a woman and her family well throughout their work together. The vignette was written to encapsulate an experience of birth that, for me, is the essence of midwifery, namely the relationship between the woman and her midwife. This is something that I experienced more as an independent and self-employed midwife than in any other area of my midwifery career. In the vignette I am in the background of the birth as it unfurls. The relationship that I had already built up with Beth enhanced my ability to assess her well-being and that of her baby. I believe that with this relationship established, it becomes possible to observe and assess the progress of labour on many of the interconnected levels of human experience. I also believe that when you get to know a woman and her family throughout her pregnancy, not only does this impact on how you relate to her in labour – it also serves to enhance the postpartum support you can provide,

> Independent Midwives are fully qualified midwives who have chosen to work outside the NHS in a self-employed capacity. Independent midwives fully support the principles of the NHS and are currently working to ensure that all women can access 'gold standard' of care in the future.
>
> *(IMUK 2013)*

Midwives do not have to work within the NHS (National Health Service) and there are a significant number of midwives who are members of IMUK or have chosen to work in private hospitals, birth centres and clinics or as self-employed midwives offering a range of services such as antenatal and postnatal care, breastfeeding support, and counselling. Many independent and non-NHS midwives are also trained in a range of complementary therapies and use these to enhance the midwifery care that they can provide.

In this chapter the term non-NHS refers to all midwives who either work for a private organisation or who are self-employed; independent midwives belong to IMUK (which was originally known as the Independent Midwives Association or the IMA). Being self-employed presents both advantages and challenges for midwives, who will have worked within the NHS either as qualified midwives or as part of their midwifery education. Since this book was first published the situation for non-NHS and independent midwives has undergone a radical shift. By 2009 the majority of non-NHS and independent midwives worked completely outside the NHS as most were unable to secure honorary contracts of employment (although the situation did vary across Britain) and they were also unable to obtain professional indemnity insurance (PII) for intrapartum care. This meant that the majority of our clients were booked for homebirths, or for antenatal and postnatal midwifery care and the non-NHS midwife would mainly act as a birthing partner if the birth was planned to take place in hospital. At this time, there were estimated to be approximately 200 independent midwives in the United Kingdom (UK), the majority of whom are members of the Independent Midwives UK (IMUK). It was unclear how many midwives were self-employed but not IMUK members.

The Nursing and Midwifery Council (NMC 2013) have stated that the UK government has recently consulted on legislation which will result in PII becoming mandatory for all health care professionals. This meant that from October 2013 all nurses and midwives would be required to have indemnity insurance to register with the NMC; at the time of writing, full implementation of this has not occurred. The need to hold an indemnity arrangement will also become a mandatory requirement of the NMC Code. This has radically changed the future for non-NHS, independent midwives and the women who use their services.

Although this legislation will cover all professional groups, it is the non-NHS and independent midwives who wish to provide complete continuity of care who have been most affected. No insurance means that they cannot register and if they are not registered they can no longer practise in the completely holistic, woman centred way that they strive for.

It could be argued that this change in legislation is one of the biggest assaults on autonomous practice since midwifery was first professionalised in the UK in 1902. Non-NHS and independent midwives have mounted campaigns to highlight their plight and have been single minded in their search for both a solution and insurance. van der Kooy (2013) has identified how IMUK has changed and developed to embrace the new health care politics of the twenty first century in an effort to find ways in which to secure professional indemnity for independent midwives. IMUK is moving towards Social Franchising for Midwives to enable midwives to set up practices which will be able to access both NHS contracts and self-funding clients. Other non-NHS midwives have looked at different types of social enterprise schemes which will enable them to obtain insurance and become sustainable in the rapidly changing health care climate. For those midwives who do not want to go down the routes already mentioned the future is very challenging and, at the time of writing, October 2013 is looming very close. The insurance issues have forced midwives (frequently with their clients beside them) to engage with government ministers and health care bodies in a sustained campaign to preserve a unique and precious service. Whilst the final position remains uncertain it is undeniable that the future of non–NHS and independent midwifery will be radically different.

All of these midwives could probably give a very different rationale for their decisions to work in a non-NHS capacity and, probably differing accounts of their practice experiences. Naturally, I can only write directly of my own experiences of independent midwifery; however, it may be possible to suggest one shared factor amongst this very diverse group of midwives – namely that they are passionate about the desire to establish their own ways of working with women. This passion is so strong that they are prepared to stand outside the NHS and wrestle with issues such as a lack of PII in order to practise what I believe to be relational midwifery. van der Hulst (1999) proposed that contemporary midwifery care is comprised of four distinct aspects, these are identified in Table 10.1.

van der Hulst's four core elements of midwifery can clearly be applied to midwifery in the UK and other settings. Reflecting back over my working life as

TABLE 10.1 van der Hulst's *Aspects of Midwifery Work* (1999)

Obstetric Technical Care	This relates to the observations, procedures and interventions that are undertaken to establish or ensure the well-being of the mother and baby.
Risk Selection	In the majority of maternity care systems women's care is based on a selection process that identifies potential or actual risk status of the mother and baby. Risk selection involves the midwife using screening processes and then referring the woman on as deemed appropriate within the system the midwife is working in.
Social Environment of the Client	Here midwives tailor their working activities to take into account the psychosocial, emotional and spiritual needs of the women they work with. For this to work successfully midwives need to move beyond a purely medicalised approach to care and view women as women with distinct individual needs.
Relational Care	Good midwifery care depends upon the establishment of a trusting relationship between the woman and the midwife. The key elements of this relationship are based upon the recognition that it is an equal partnership based upon empowerment, openness and self-activation on behalf of both sides of the partnership.

a midwife I can see how these four aspects have been present in all the different midwifery settings in which I have worked. So far, my independent practice has been the only midwifery experience that gave me enough time and space to synergise van der Hulst's four aspects within my clinical life. Like all midwives I need good technical skills and the ability to assess well-being. However, when I work directly with women, rather than with an institution, these aspects harmonise with the considerations of the individual woman and the relationship of mutual trust that we aim to establish. Fahy (2012) identifies midwifery as primarily a profession that should be founded on the relationships between women and their midwives. These professional relationships recognise the importance of a woman's health needs and expectations and the right of women to self-determination.

Being non-NHS or independent means you often have a different relationship with your clients, one where the contract of employment is usually negotiated directly between the woman and the midwife. I would argue that the intimate nature of this working relationship is a result of the partnership it engenders. However, when the midwife is an employee of an institution, the ensuing relationship between a woman and her midwife is mediated by the midwife's contract to that institution and therefore by the nature of that institution and the complexity of the service that it endeavours to supply. It is hard to estimate how the changes in non-NHS midwifery practice will impact on this relationship.

However, it can be argued that the common result of this relational triangle is an imbalance in what van der Hulst has identified as the main aspects of midwifery work. Reflecting back on my own working experiences, I would suggest that van der Hulst's imbalance represents the challenges faced by midwives working in large institutional settings where there is arguably an emphasis on technical care and risk selection, to the potential detriment of those aspects concerned with relational care and the social environment of the client. Lawrence Beech and Phipps (2008) have proposed that in our contemporary society we do not fully recognise the significance and impact of birth on women's emotional well-being and the subsequent transition into motherhood. They go on to suggest that this lack of recognition is reflected within the systems that serve our birthing culture.

> It is generally expected that the woman should be satisfied with the birth of a live baby, irrespective of the way the birth happened. The failure to acknowledge and address the mother's experiences leaves too many women with traumatizing memories, rather than positive and empowering ones. Often this is because we have allowed systems to develop that interfere with the birth process.
>
> *(Lawrence Beech and Phipps 2008:69)*

Independent and non-NHS practice has the potential to provide a way of practising midwifery that addresses some of the above issues. It has enabled me to practise midwifery in a way that allowed a balance between the different aspects of my midwifery work.

A personal journey towards autonomy

As I gained experience of working as a midwife I wanted to have more control in organising my working life. My perception of what independent practice entailed was rooted in my personal feminist philosophy. Kaufmann (2004) states that a feminist midwifery profession:

> Supports and values the women who work within it, asking them to work in solidarity with each other and with the women in their care in order to help all women have the birth experience they deserve.
>
> *(Kaufmann 2004: 9)*

The decision to work independently can be hedged with many issues, not least the move from being an employee to becoming self-employed, or moving from student status within NHS institutions to qualified status on the outside of those same institutions. Anxiety about being unable to earn a living can act as a deterrent to starting up in practice. Hobbs (1997) advised that initially midwives should consider how they plan to support themselves until they have clients booked. Starting up a practice involves not just establishing a client base but also buying and maintaining equipment. Having a network of other experienced midwives to call upon for information, support and advice was invaluable for me as I worked out what I needed and where to obtain it. Although there are only a few independent midwives in Scotland I never felt unsupported. My experiences have always been that other midwives are generous with their time, advice and support. I have found that the majority of independent and self-employed midwives I have got to know over the years are very good at liaising both with each other and other midwives and health professionals.

Of all the health professions, midwifery remains the most heavily regulated. Each time I met with prospective clients we discussed in depth the issues of insurance, midwifery supervision and professional responsibility. Such discussions form the bedrock of any future working relationships and also reinforce my concepts of what it means to be an autonomous practitioner.

Autonomous practice and client choice

The NHS operates a comprehensive maternity care system designed to support a large and diverse population; as such it would not be unreasonable to wonder why women would chose to book with an independent midwife. After all why pay for a service that is widely available free of charge? My experience of being self-employed echoes that of many of my colleagues in that women seek out an independent midwife because the service that they are looking for is not available to them in their local area. Frequently women want continuity of midwife and to know the midwife who will be with them when they go into labour. Women will therefore choose an independent or self-employed midwife because the alternative might be an unknown midwife from a large team of midwives. The importance for women in labour of already knowing their midwife is often dismissed by sceptics who claim that all women really want is someone who is skilled and kind. Pilley Edwards' (2000) study of women planning homebirths highlighted the importance of knowing and therefore being able to trust the midwife who was with you in labour. In the study women reported fears about being transferred into hospital unnecessarily. For some women this fear was made worse by the fact that they did not really know their midwives. Where midwives had been able to provide continuity, women perceived their relationship as providing personal support and professional competencies. This blend of personal and professional was seen as crucial for the mother–midwife interaction and achievable only when there was continuity in the interaction between the woman and her midwife.

Women may also decide to book with an independent or self-employed midwife if they experience difficulty in accessing specific sets of skills such as vaginal breech birth, home VBAC (vaginal birth after caesarean), homebirth or home water birth. From my own experiences and from the experiences of my colleagues a significant number of women will seek out alternative midwifery care because of their previous birth experiences and a subsequent desire to have more control over what will happen to them in their current pregnancy.

Independent and self-employed practice is criticised for providing a limited and potentially elitist service because women have to be able to pay for their midwifery care. There is arguably an element of truth in this accusation, as non-NHS midwifery care is not free and therefore it is not equally available to all women. However there is a broad spectrum of women who access non-NHS midwives and many midwives try and adopt flexible systems of payment and barter.

Independent and non-NHS midwifery is one of a number of ways in which the autonomy of the midwife is clearly manifested. As autonomous practitioners midwives can work as self-employed upon the point of qualifying and registration. This ability of midwives to establish a self-employed working practice could be cited as evidence of the autonomy of the midwifery profession. However it is the very autonomy of most non-NHS and independent midwives that can sometimes appear to place them at odds with the contemporary health environment. Working outside a clear management structure also places most non-NHS and independent midwives in a potentially difficult position – how do you deal with or discipline a midwife who has no manager to report to? It would appear that the answer to this would be to use midwifery supervision (see Chapter 6) as a quasi-management tool and then report the midwife to the NMC (Nursing and Midwifery Council). The NMC is the regulatory body for nursing and midwifery and as such has a responsibility for any disciplinary or investigatory procedures involving registrants. Being investigated by your professional body is a daunting prospect for any midwife, but for a non-NHS or independent midwife this can be particularly difficult. If you are suspended from practice pending investigation you are effectively prevented from earning your living through midwifery. If there are no charges proved, it is virtually impossible to claim back any lost earnings. Wagner (2004) writing about what he has termed a 'global witch hunt' states:

It is no coincidence that 70 per cent of the accused in my sample are midwives, all in independent practice where they are not under the immediate control of doctors. Fear of being investigated by authorities is a strong deterrent to independent midwives.

(Wagner 2004:36)

Working independently can mean being perceived as an 'outsider'. Different hospitals have different ways of organising themselves and it can be challenging to negotiate systems that are not always apparent. As an outsider it can be difficult communicating with other health professionals who may not understand alternative ways of working or who choose to display outward hostility towards either non-NHS or independent midwives or to their clients. The following vignette relates to the transfer of a client, Jo, to hospital following a long labour, demonstrating the move from a holistic perspective of birth into a completely different setting. Jo was transferred from a setting corresponding to van der Hulst's concept of relational care into a setting that could be identified as having risk selection and obstetrical technical care dominating over any other considerations.

VIGNETTE 2

Arrival on labour ward was as difficult as the strained nature of the transfer phone call had intimated. Faces peered at us over the midwives' desk as we came in, no real welcome, just staring. Once we were in a delivery room we were joined by two midwives, one friendly, one openly hostile. Unfortunately for Jo and Tony, the friendly midwife went away and we were left with the hostile one. It was hard to tell whether the disapproval was aimed at, Jo, Tony, myself, or at all of us.

While we waited for a doctor a range of sniping comments were directed at the three of us.

The decision to transfer in was accompanied by a sense of loss for a planned birth experience and a sense of trepidation and vulnerability over what to expect next. Given these circumstances Jo's reception on delivery suite did nothing to alleviate any of her concerns and in fact reinforced her fears.

Reflecting on Jo's birth experience outlined in Vignette 2, I would suggest that the hostility we experienced when we transferred in had more to do with the underlying clash of systems and philosophies of care than with any particular individual involved within the situation. Davis-Floyd and Sargent (1997) would contextualize this within the technocratic framework of modern childbirth. For non-NHS or independent midwives it represents the difficulty of mediating between relational midwifery and institutional midwifery in an environment where you are treated as an outsider and you move from being midwife to birth supporter. Leap (2000) writes that when women need to give birth with the support of obstetric technology our active recognition of their courage and endurance has potentially empowering consequences for the early transition into motherhood. Kirkham (2000) identified that organisational and medical care aims should incorporate the aims of individual women. However, she observes that there is invariably a tension between the aims of the individual and the generalised provision of care. For the non-NHS or independent midwife working on the outside of a system, yet still connected to it by the needs of her clients, this tension is often very apparent. Jo, Tony and I perceived their time on labour ward as alienating and disempowering. Fortunately for Jo and Tony the negative perceptions of the hospital system were counterbalanced by their positive experiences with the midwives on the postnatal ward.

For non-NHS practice to work well for both midwives and women it is essential to be able to work with other health professionals in responding to the changing needs of women during their childbearing experiences.

VIGNETTE 3

When we arrived the staff were reassuring and friendly. The midwife I handed over to went through the notes and listened to what Bronwyn and Iain had to say, making a point of finding out what they had written in their birth plan. When the consultant came in to see Bronwyn she was very friendly and interested, again asking them about their plans for the labour. The atmosphere in the room was positive, calm and caring. Ewan was delivered by forceps, and the consultant made sure that Iain was still able to cut the cord and that Bronwyn had Ewan straight away for a first breastfeed.

Bronwyn did not have the birth she planned, but she later commented that she felt satisfied with the decisions that were made and with the care she received. She had a known midwife with her all the time, and when she transferred into hospital she felt involved in all the decision-making, supported by everyone involved. As Bronwyn's midwife I felt that there was a partnership between the couple, the hospital staff and myself. There were no underlying care conflicts or ideology clashes, but rather a co-operative approach to ensure the best outcome.

Working as an independent midwife made me remember why I wanted to be a midwife in the first place. I wanted a job that would let me use my heart and mind rather than one where I had to sell my soul just to survive. I firmly believe that the future of midwifery is being held in the balance whilst a small group of midwives challenge the seeming lack of political will to address insurance issues which will leave women with fewer choices.

References

Davis-Floyd, R. and Sargent, C.F. (eds.) (1997) *Childbirth and Authoritative Knowledge: Cross Cultural Perspectives.* Berkeley: University of California Press.

Fahy, K. (2012) 'What is woman centred care and why does it matter?' *Women and Birth* 25(4): 149–51.

Hobbs, L. (1997) *The Independent Midwife: A Guide to Independent Midwifery*, 2nd edition. Practice Hale: Books for Midwives.

IMUK (2013) Independent Midwives UK. http://www.independentmidwives.org.uk. Accessed July 2013.

Kaufmann, T. (2004) 'Introducing feminism', in M. Stewart (ed.) *Pregnancy, Birth and Maternity Care: Feminist Perspectives.* Edinburgh: Books for Midwives Press, Elsevier, pp. 1–10.

Kirkham, M. (ed.) (2000) *The Midwife–Mother Relationship.* Basingstoke: Macmillan Press Limited.

Lawrence Beech, B.A and Phipps, B. (2008) 'Normal birth: women's stories', in S. Downe (ed.) *Normal Birth: Evidence and Debate*, 2nd edition. Edinburgh: Churchill Livingstone Elsevier, pp. 67–79.

Leap, N. (2000) 'The less we do the more we give', in M. Kirkham (ed.) *The Midwife–Mother Relationship.* Basingstoke: Macmillan Press Limited, pp. 1–18.

NMC (2013) *Statement on Professional Indemnity Insurance.* http://www.nmc-uk.org/ Registration/Professional-indemnity-insurance/. Accessed 4 July 2013.

Pilley Edwards, N. (2000) 'Women planning homebirths: their own views on their relationships with midwives', in M. Kirkham (ed.) *The Midwife–Mother Relationship.* Basingstoke: Macmillan Press Limited, pp. 55–91.

van der Hulst, L.A.M. (1999) 'Dutch midwives: relational care and birth location'. *Health and Social Care in the Community* (7): 242–47.

van der Kooy, B. (2013) 'Social franchising for midwives'. *Midwifery Matters* 137(summer): 6–7.

Wagner, M. (2004) 'A global witch hunt'. *Midwifery Matters* 100(Spring): 36.

Commentary

Nessa's chapter opens with a vignette which I am fairly sure must have touched the heartstrings of all readers. It sounds like an ideal birth for the woman concerned, her family and the two midwives involved. However very quickly thereafter she moves on to explain that while such a scenario is the high point of independent midwifery, there are currently many low points taking up independent midwives' time and energy and causing some to give up independent practice and return to working in hospitals. Almost 20 years ago the midwifery professional organisation balloted its members (mostly midwives practising in hospitals) on the topic of financial support, through providing professional indemnity insurance, for independent midwives. As a result of that ballot being strongly against hospital midwives supporting independent midwives, the organisation withdrew its financial subsidies. The current crisis has been provoked by new legislations being enacted in the European parliament, the result of which is that all health professionals must have professional indemnity insurance, thereby placing another financial burden on independent midwives (this is also discussed in Chapter 4).

Nessa reflects on a further two vignettes, neither of which reflect the ideal outcome for women but both of which have a very different effect on the midwife. In cases of transfer from the home into hospital it is almost a lottery as to how the woman and her independent midwife will be received. Interestingly in my own PhD (Fleming 1994) one New Zealand midwife who had been a senior midwife in a labour ward for 16 years experienced a similarly hostile greeting and even had her competence questioned when less than a month after moving into independent practice she had to transfer a woman to her previous place of employment. Such a situation is also evident in the research currently being carried out in Switzerland (Meyer *et al.*, 2013) where both women and midwives report on positive and negative experiences.

References

Fleming, V. (1994) 'Partnership, politics and power. Feminist expectations of midwifery practice'. PhD thesis. Massey University.

Meyer, Y. and Pehlke-Milde, J. (2013) 'Verlegung: Interim Report'. Presented at the Conference of German Obstetricians and Gynaecologists, Berlin, December 2013.

11

A MALE MIDWIFE'S PERSPECTIVE

Denis Walsh

VIGNETTE

Sally was a friend I had met through my local church. She had suffered from ME for over a decade, during which time she was unemployed, though she was highly qualified. I lost touch with her when I moved to another part of the city but had heard that she had married in her late 30s. Then, out of the blue I got a phone call from her to say that she was pregnant and asked if I would be her midwife. I was working as team leader midwife and had begun to develop a small personal caseload. I enthusiastically agreed. Sally wanted a home water-birth which I was very happy to support her with, though she was 39 and still suffered with ME whose main symptoms were excessive fatigue and lethargy. The obstetrician did not raise any objections, though I knew she was pessimistic that the labour would be straightforward. I did all the antenatal care at Sally's home and observed over the course of the pregnancy a remission in her symptoms of ME. She was genuinely excited about the baby and birth and went into labour on a bright sunny morning in May. After a reasonably quick first stage and a 3-hour second stage she gave birth to a robust baby boy in the pool. It was a magic moment. The French doors to the garden were open, the sun was streaming through and we could hear children playing in the adjacent park during the labour. She did not lack energy during the labour, pushed with great gusto and had an uneventful postnatal period. She was a confident, instinctive mother. I remember driving home after the birth, feeling proud and elated that I had facilitated a birth that I am sure would have been inter-ventionist in a maternity hospital. In the 1990s, an elderly primigravida with a history of a debilitating condition would not have been seen as a good candidate for a home birth. For me, it was the realisation of an ideal regarding what being a midwife was all about: personalised, supportive, empathic care for a woman according to her needs and her choices. I had not witnessed a medical event, I had witnessed one of nature's marvels – human childbirth in the perfect setting. She had done it and I was the privileged bystander. To this day, I understand her experience as a healing one. The woman she was at the beginning of pregnancy was not the confident mother she became. She had gone on a transformatory journey and it was beautiful to witness.

Though I had been a midwife about 5 years before having this experience, I don't think I had really understood what being a midwife was truly about until that experience. I had been drawn to midwifery because of the autonomy of the role and the fact that its focus was not illness. In my early years of practice, exclusively in a large maternity hospital, I found that autonomy hard to realise. In addition, though everyone talked about normal birth, most of what I saw and experienced was not normal. I was living with considerable dissonance and during those years my practice was mostly about resistance to the biomedical model and the steady accumulation of physiological birth skills within the relative privacy of the birth room. That prepared me for the opportunity outlined above. However, the experience of Sally's birth reordered my priorities, for the experience was not about my autonomy, but Sally's, and not about my skills but hers. It was the first time I really understood what 'being with woman' was all about and its impact was profound. Since that time I have pursued a teaching and research career that gave me the opportunity to research this area in the context of birth centres and to challenge midwives to critically reflect on their intrapartum practice through workshops and seminars.

Aspects of lived experience of being a male midwife

During my training, I rationalised that what I 'brought to the table' as a male midwife was no different to what the childless female midwife brought: their humanity, compassion, empathy and interpersonal skills. It was not until I started to read feminist critiques of childbirth and feminist literature more widely that I realised this was a rather naive position. Of course gender mediates care encounters and no matter how sensitive one is to women's responses, just being male can imbue scenarios with power differentials that disadvantage women. This awareness is so important that I now believe that knowledge of feminist critiques of childbirth is not an optional extra for a male midwife. Along with Schacht and Ewing (1997), I believe it forms one of four key challenges if a male midwife is to practise with integrity. The other challenges are to consider reflexively what he as an individual, and men as a group, do to oppress women; to consider ways to reject traditional notions of masculinity that are oppressive to others and to consider feminist values and ethics as a referent for personal practice. Finally, Schacht and Ewing urge male practitioners to consider ways to place women's needs as equal to or greater than his own. I have found these considerations helpful in approaching and understanding what it means for me to be a midwife, to care for women and to work with female midwifery colleagues.

Pragmatically, I apply this in practice by having sensitive antennae to women's discomfort zone when I turn up as their carer. Often they may state their preference for a female attendant but even if I can detect non-verbal behaviours that display this discomfort, I will offer to be replaced with a female colleague. Male midwife colleagues take an even more proactive position by requesting female midwives to inform women in advance that they have a male colleague on the team and that it is acceptable to desist from his care. I did not take this route because I thought that it might be interpreted by women that I was also uncomfortable. As I was the first male midwife to train and work locally, I wanted to communicate that I was at ease with the intimacy of the midwife/woman relationship. Because of this desire I prioritise rapport building with women when I first meet them. I approach the task of forming interpersonal relationships by having an informal, easy-going style. Personally, I see the relationship as akin to what Page (1995) called a 'professional friendship', mutually disclosing as friends would when this seems appropriate. I am not uncomfortable with the expression of emotions that regularly occurs in birth, nor the use of touch to support or empathise with women. Touch, though, has to be measured and considered. I would not, for example, hold a woman in an embrace beyond a brief hug, though I know female midwives who do this with great effect depending on the situation. As a rule of thumb I don't undertake vaginal examinations unless the woman has a companion with her and I use a non-touch technique when advising on positioning for breast-feeding. Trust and rapport are very important for care encounters in pregnancy and childbirth and, for this reason, I prefer models of care that give space for their development. With those in place, the appropriate backdrop for intimate examinations exists. For these reasons, chaperoning by another member of staff is not required in my view.

One aspect I am regularly asked about in relation to caring for women in labour is how do their male partners react. Rarely, in my experience, do men object to me being the midwife. When they do, it is usually because of cultural or religious prohibitions or, less commonly, because they dislike their partners being cared for by a man. As when women show some disquiet, when this occurs with men, I immediately withdraw. Once, I had built a good rapport with a woman over several hours of labour (she had her mother with her) until her partner turned up near the end of the labour. When I was relieved for a break, he told the midwife that he did not want me attending his partner, so I withdrew. After the baby was born, I went in to see her (the partner had left by then) and she was crying. She said she was mortified at his earlier actions and thought it would have really upset me. I reassured her that was not the case but clearly he was unable to cope with having a male attendant. Usually, I have a very good relationship with a male birth companion and take the time to get to know him by seeking common areas to converse on. Though this probably puts him at ease, it is not always helpful for the birth room atmosphere. Conversation and attention diverted to others in the birth room can be distracting for the woman and could compromise my own observation and connection with her. Generally I take those opportunities in early labour but not as labour progresses. The other dimension in relationship to male partners that is interesting occurs in couple childbirth preparation classes. Over the years, together with female colleagues, we have split the classes on gender lines at particular junctures and I have facilitated the men talking about their experiences of the antenatal period. Gradually they start to share worries and concerns, often with respect to relationship tensions. These sessions have been well evaluated by men and expose unmet needs in this group which latterly the Fatherhood Institute (2008) have taken forward.

As good as a female midwife?

What has troubled me more over the years is whether I can support women in labour as well as my female colleagues. A male midwife friend eventually left the profession and one of the aspects he particularly struggled with was how patronising he felt when verbally encouraging women through the intensity of labour. Knowing he could never share this experience made him feel his words were patronising and paternalistic. Of course one could argue that childless female midwives may feel the same but at least they share the same reproductive biology. As I read about intuition and heard stories of highly intuitive midwives, I was concerned that there was some female reservoir of wisdom and insight that I could never tap into as a man. Around the same time, feminist scholarship was beginning to challenge gender essentialism (Annandale and Clark 1996) as postmodern ideas were explored. Postmodern perspectives challenge taken-for-granted assumptions behind discourses like the biomedical model, capitalism, democracy etc. In the same way they challenge the idea that men and women think and act differently (Gray 1992), arguing that differences are socially constructed and serve to reinforce stereotypes and roles. This opened up the possibility that intuitive skills could be modelled or accrued through mentoring and observation and were not fixed as female-only characteristics. More recently, Moberg and Petersson (2006) has written that oxytocin, a key hormone secreted by labouring women that initiates and progresses labour, is also secreted by men, especially through compassionate care and therapeutic touch. This suggests that male companions or carers in labour can be a facilitatory presence. Recent research on the effectiveness of the child's father as a birth companion supports this (Kainz *et al.* 2010).

Much of what might be considered characteristics of good care – listening skills, empathy, kindness, sensitivity to individual needs, up-to-date knowledge, clinical skills – could be argued are generic across genders. There is an additional and important dimension that links to intuitive care but is not the same as that which has been popularised in contemporary management and self-help literature – emotional intelligence (Goleman 1996). My own research into the work of staff in birth centres suggests that birth attendants there utilise emotional intelligence in the care of women to great effect. I hypothesised this as matrescent (becoming mother) care that is a subtle blend of comforting, encouraging, enabling and leaving alone (Walsh 2006). Hunter (2005) and Dahlen *et al.* (2010) also write about the importance of emotional work by midwives. This kind of sensitivity is related to having a high degree of self-awareness, competence and confidence in relationships and being comfortable with the intimacy and embodied aspects of childbirth. All of these are unlikely to be the preserve of women only.

Apart from positive feedback from women about the effectiveness of my care, these ideas have helped sustain me in clinical practice.

Conflict and gender

What I did not anticipate in my career as a midwife was conflict with male obstetricians that would significantly influence my decision to leave full-time practice. Again, feminist critique has illuminated gender games in the workplace, in particular the doctor/nurse game in health: the female nurse has a great idea to improve care but to implement it she has to sell it to the male doctor so that he takes ownership of it (Sweet & Norman 1995). Part of her selling technique may involve flirtatious behaviours and 'friendly banter'. That game has strong resonances with what I have observed in maternity units but it has obvious limitations when the midwife is male. I was told an amended version by a male health service manager. He recommended building a 'blokey rapport' with male consultants (conversations around sport, cars, drinking exploits) so that you are on first name terms. The next step is to present new ideas as a solution to existing problems so that the doctor's life will be easier. He can then get on with his job of expert clinician without management interference.

These strategies have more than a touch of compromising one's integrity and buying into unhelpful power relationships and hierarchies which remain unchallenged. At the extreme end of these manipulative behaviours and compliance with the status quo may be bullying and intimidation that is allowed to continue. For all of these reasons, I never took this path and, maybe as a consequence, encountered conflict regularly with some male obstetricians.

Territorial disputes

Complicating gender politics in maternity care are historical professional struggles between obstetrics and midwifery. These transcend gender and are therefore played out between female midwives and obstetricians and male midwives and male obstetricians, as described above. My own view is that a lot of these conflicts are accentuated by the context of institutional care in large busy hospitals. Where space is made for building trust and mutual understanding, a true partnership in care can emerge and a positive inter-disciplinary environment can flourish. Along with Downe *et al.* (2007), I don't believe pigeon-holing obstetricians or midwives as anti or pro normal birth is helpful or even accurate and the most creative and best maternity services exist where the common ground is shared.

Having said that, the potent effect of professional group socialisation often results in midwives who lack autonomy and the assertiveness skills to address this (Ball *et al.* 2003). Many midwives hear themselves being referred to as 'my midwives', or experts in meeting psycho-social needs but marginalised from real clinical autonomy, in their dealings with obstetricians. There are a number of strategies that I think are helpful in remedying this. One is the mandatory teaching of assertiveness skill training, using role play and reflection, for all student midwives. A second is investing in continuity models of working, based in primary care. The experience of autonomy is facilitated by the greater independent status that can be realised from a primary care base. Hand in hand with autonomy goes accountability and midwives need nurturing into accepting these twin professional responsibilities. It is only from a secure sense of one's own skill base and confidence in one's role that relationships of equality with other professional groups can be entered into. I have observed great examples of positive inter-professional working between midwives and obstetricians in recent years and these need modelling and replicating more widely. One strategic feature that would assist midwifery's self-confidence is obtaining representation in the more strategic local NHS Trust posts like clinical director or chief executive. Very senior posts in the NHS are gendered, reflecting the under-representation of women in senior management posts more broadly in society (Moore & Buttner 1997). It was very encouraging to read Byrom and Downe's (2010) paper on transformational leadership in midwifery. These are exactly the kind of posts, individuals and styles of leadership that can help the profession out of its historical inferiority to medicine.

Academic life as a male midwife

Though my exposure to feminist literature and scholarship has been since I have worked in universities, I can honestly say that, in the main, other female midwifery academics have been very welcoming and inclusive. Even those who had previously published their reservations about the entry of men into the profession have been supportive and encouraging. About 8 years ago, in the midst of doubts about my continued contribution to midwifery as a man, two experiences convinced me that I could make a worthwhile contribution. One was the reception and feedback I got from the launch of an evidence course in normal labour and birth which has subsequently been attended by over 3,000 midwives in many countries. The second was an invitation to contribute a chapter to an edited book about feminist perspectives on pregnancy and childbirth (Stewart 2003). That another midwife could think I could input into such a book was amazing. Since then, I have had one negative experience as a midwifery academic when I was misquoted in a national press article (Campbell 2009) and received a torrent of negative headlines and vindictive emails over the next month. However, alongside these, I got fantastic support from midwives who knew me and now I look back on that experience as a steep learning curve in dealing with the media. The experience helped me to realise that taking up a feminist position as a man presented a special opportunity to discuss and debate feminism's critique of western childbirth. Teaching students and presenting at conferences seem to open up stimulating debates that challenged presuppositions people had about this topic.

I currently teach a session on gender empowerment to student midwives at my university and am constantly surprised that the word 'feminism' has such negative connotations for the female students. This is despite the terrible statistic that domestic violence kills two women per week in the UK, that women continue to be under-represented in public life and that women are still paid less for the same job than their male counterparts (Banyard 2010).

I am now a strong advocate of a feminist discourse underpinning undergraduate midwifery curricula. Feminist values should be embedded and taught explicitly and the history of feminist thought and actions covered in the sociology of birth. This is because women still birth within a largely patriarchal society.

Another aspect of academic work that has been challenging is undertaking research into childbirth. Being a male researcher interviewing exclusively female research participants has raised a number of issues for me. There was a time when I thought that my gender should prohibit me from doing childbirth research. If Oakley, a pioneering feminist, struggled with the idea of researching women's experience as she debates in the thought-provoking chapter 'Interviewing women: a contradiction in terms' (Oakley 1981), then how could a man?

One of the issues was the whole notion of being a researcher first and a person second in relation to data collection and interactions with people in the field. Others with feminist sensitivities have construed this dilemma as 'faking friendship' (Duncombe & Jessop 2002) and this phrase captures the ambivalence it creates for the researcher. In the textbooks, one of the dangers of ethnographic fieldwork includes the possibility of 'going native' where identification with the observed group reaches a point where the outsider perspective is lost (Donovan 2005). I found myself dropping the researcher persona, and relating quite spontaneously and naturally. It occurred several months into fieldwork and reflected the fact that I was forming relationships with the staff and an easy familiarity was evolving. Instead of me listening and observing, I was starting to tell stories and generally reveal more of myself to them.

The challenge in these situations is to have congruence about one's authenticity and genuineness while remaining a researcher first. Achieving a sense of congruence is not just for one's own integrity but also out of respect for those being contacted in the field. Feminist writers particularly put a high value on this with their central concern to diminish power differentials between the researcher and the research participant.

Conclusion

It is interesting to speculate about the popularity of midwifery as a career option for men. I suspect that the number of men entering the profession has not changed that much since Lewis's (1991) original survey of more than 20 years ago now. It may be that because the male midwife has high visibility within the service, this results in a level of scrutiny that many men would not welcome. Or that the nature of the work is simply unappealing, though this begs the question as to why obstetrics and gynaecology remain relatively popular with male doctors.

High visibility can be an advantage if the male midwife is popular with staff and clients but equally, perceived short-comings precede you wherever you go. Early on in my training I was greeted once with: 'I heard you were quite normal'!

I have no regrets about my decision to become a midwife. It has provided some of the most memorable experiences of my life and through it I have met many remarkable people, both fellow midwives and mothers. Of course I have concerns about the medicalisation of childbirth, the semi-autonomous but not often enough full autonomy of our role and the effects of an institutional model on women. However, the privilege of witnessing and attending physiological birth and latterly, the opportunity to research, teach and discuss childbirth with committed midwifery practitioners and academics sustains me.

References

Annandale, E. and Clark, J. (1996) 'What is gender? Feminist theory and the sociology of human reproduction'. *Sociology of Health and Illness* 18: 17–44.

Ball, L., Curtis, P. and Kirkham, M. (2003) *Why do midwives leave?* London: Royal College of Midwives.

Banyard, K. (2010) *The Equality Illusion: The Truth About Women and Men Today*. London: Faber & Faber.

Byrom, S. and Downe, S. (2010) '"She sort of shines": midwives' accounts of "good" midwifery and "good" leadership'. *Midwifery* 26(1): 126–37.

Campbell, D. (2009) 'It's good for women to suffer the pain of a natural birth'. *Observer*, May 29th.

Dahlen, H.G., Barclay, L.M. and Homer, C.S.E. (2010) 'The novice birthing: theorising first-time mothers' experiences of birth at home and in hospital in Australia'. *Midwifery* 26(1): 53–63.

Donovan, P. (2005) 'Ethnography', in E. Cluett and R. Bluff (eds), *Principles and Practice of Research in Midwifery*. London: Bailliere Tindall.

Downe, S., Mckeown, M. *et al.* (2007) 'The UCLan community engagement and service user support (Comensus) project: valuing authenticity, making space for emergence'. *Health Expectations* 10(4): 392–406.

Duncombe, J. and Jessop, J. (2002) '"Doing rapport" and the ethics of "faking friendship"', in M. Mauthner, M. Birch, J. Jessop, and T. Miller (eds), *Ethics in Qualitative Research*. London: Sage Publications, pp. 107–22.

Fatherhood Institute (2008) *The Dad Deficit: The Missing Piece of the Maternity Jigsaw*. London: DHA Communications.

Goleman, D. (1996) *Emotional Intelligence*. London: Bloomsbury.

Gray, J. (1992) *Men are from Mars, Women are from Venus*. London: Bloomsbury.

Hunter, B. (2005) 'Emotion work and boundary maintenance in hospital-based midwifery'. *Midwifery* 21(3): 253–66.

Kainz, G., Eliasson, M. and von Post, I. (2010) 'The child's father, an important person for the mother's well-being during the childbirth: A hermeneutic study'. *Health Care for Women International* 31(7):621–35.

Lewis, P. (1991) 'Men in midwifery: their experiences as students and practitioners', in S. Robinson and A. Thomson (eds), *Midwives, Research and Childbirth*. London: Chapman & Hall.

Moberg, K.U. and Petersson, M. (2006) 'Antistress, well-being, empathy and social support', in B.B. Arnetz and R. Ekman (eds), *Stress in Health and Disease*. Weinheim, FRG: Wiley-VCH Verlag GmbH and Co. KgaA.

Moore, D. and Buttner, E. (1997) *Moving Beyond the Glass Ceiling*. London: Sage Publications.

Oakley, A. (1981) 'Interviewing women: a contradiction in terms', in H. Roberts (ed.), *Doing Feminist Research*. London: Routledge.

Page, L. (1995) 'Putting principles into practice', in L. Page (ed.) *Effective Group Practice in Midwifery: Working with Women*. Oxford: Blackwell Science.

Schacht, S. and Ewing, S. (1997) 'The many paths of feminism: can men travel any of them?' *Journal of Gender Studies* 6(2): 159–76.

Sweet, S. and Norman, I. (1995) 'The nurse-doctor relationship: a selective literature review'. *Journal of Advanced Nursing* 22: 165–70.

Stewart, M. (2003) *Pregnancy, Birth and Maternity Care: Feminist Perspectives*. London: BfM.

Walsh, D. (2006) '"Nesting" and "matrescence": distinctive features of a free-standing birth centre'. *Midwifery* 22(3): 228–39.

Commentary

With his title alone Denis highlights the notion of 'being different', a notion he goes on to explore and to challenge. As he points out, a man who practises midwifery is still rare in the UK, his adopted country, and in other European countries figures are similar. In times where equality between the sexes is encouraged it appears midwifery is not attractive to men. In the late 1970s when legislation changed in the UK permitting men to enter midwifery education, it became reasonably popular to do so for a few years. These, however, were the times when a 'second certificate' was necessary to gain promotion in general nursing and the availability of midwifery widened the options for men. Thankfully these times have changed and those entering midwifery do so generally because they wish to practise midwifery rather than receive promotion in another field. However, in some countries, notably those in the Middle East, men are prohibited from applying for midwifery education at all. Perhaps in keeping with their strict segregation of the sexes in health care this decision is right for those countries because in nursing over 50 per cent of students are now men. This means that 50 per cent of the graduates can provide care to both men and women and the other

50 per cent to men only. Of the women who are nurses, many go on to have their own children leaving a potentially huge gap in qualified nurses able to provide health care for women. This will not happen in midwifery at the present time.

What does it mean to be different? It would be possible here to have made comparisons between women as airline pilots for example where I have heard it said 'would you like her to be flying if she was pre-menstrual?' Rather than dwelling on such differences, however, Denis has written eloquently about the meaning of being a midwife striving to provide a physiological birth experience for women in his care. He highlights some of the positive and negative experiences and how he has addressed them and as progressed in his chosen profession . . . that of midwifery.

12

DO WOMEN CARE IF THEIR MIDWIFE HAS HAD CHILDREN?

A reflection on changing my mind

Carrie McIntosh

'Do you have children yourself?'

A question I'm sure every midwife reading this can identify with. Why is it that the pregnant or new mother asks this of her midwife? Are they just making conversation? Mander (2009) suggests that this is unlikely as there are far too many other things going on during this time in her life; it is more likely there is some kind of agenda, purpose or issue requiring resolution. Is it, then, that the woman places credence on the midwife's skills depending on her answer? Alternatively, does having had children make you a better midwife? It's an interesting topic, which has sparked many a debate. My observation, not surprisingly, is that many childless or childfree midwives will argue that it makes no difference. I have to admit that my opinions have done a U–turn over the years. I reflect here on how this happened.

VIGNETTE

Living in an affluent area, Valerie was a career-minded woman who, by her own admission, had left childbearing to later in life so she could establish her career. Like many first-time parents, this couple was anxious to know they were doing everything right. In response to my question about how their first night after coming home had been, she picked up her notepad and reeled off a detailed hour-by-hour account of the baby's feeding and nappy changes. Finally, she anxiously asked 'does that all sound ok?' I reassured her that it all sounded perfectly normal. Probing further though, I smiled and asked 'but how were *you*?' Trying to gauge how she and her partner felt about being at home

---

together as a family, Valerie laughed, her shoulders dropped visibly and she relaxed, replying 'knackered!'. The visit took some time as they both had a lot of questions, ranging from how often and how long the baby should feed, down to what brand of nappies did I think were the best.

I answered all their questions patiently while trying to convince them that a lot of parenting decisions were based on trial and error and that they must try to learn to trust their own instincts as parents. Books and health professionals do not have all the answers. Valerie laughed again and asked the inevitable question – 'Do you have children yourself?'. 'Yes' I replied, 'I have three'. 'Aaaah' was her response 'I can tell. You just sound so knowledgeable – as if you're talking from experience'. Valerie went on to tell me that the midwife who had provided her antenatal care had been very young. They had also asked her a lot of questions but confided that they hadn't actually trusted anything she had told them. They felt that her age and the fact that she didn't have any children gave less credence to the information she gave – 'it sounded like she was quoting from a book, not from experience'. Valerie went on to remark how much happier she felt having spoken with me who had answered their questions 'properly'.

I can't deny that I felt proud at their praise. For the rest of the day I walked around with a little smile, thinking 'I did a good job there'. Then I started to reflect. Was I the font of all knowledge and did this other midwife have a long way to go both in years and experience before women would trust her? Of course not.

I thought back to my experiences as a first-time mother. Aged 25 and prior to becoming a midwife, I was expecting my first baby. I admit to not being the belligerent questioning radical I am now. My pregnancy knowledge comprised what I read in the literature given out at the booking-in appointment. I assumed I would be told all I needed to know by my GP and the midwives at the antenatal classes. I don't think I even knew what midwives did. All my antenatal care was carried out by my GP – I didn't know there was an alternative. I had met a lovely midwife who took blood at the booking-in appointment and remarked that she'd better be prepared for me to faint as I usually did at such times. She chatted to me, finally announcing 'That's you done!' I was so surprised, I hadn't felt a thing. I was impressed that this midwife was the first person to take my blood without me ending up a heap on the floor.

Five months then passed before I met a midwife again and it was at my first antenatal class. I was so surprised and pleased that the class was taken by the same midwife, who I'll call Barbara (not her real name). After introducing herself to the group of 20 or so, she proceeded to chat about what we could expect when coming into the hospital to have our babies. Barbara explained she had four children and, although this was 16 years ago, I clearly remember the moment she said those words – I was sold. I already idolised this woman for her skills with a needle, but now I knew she was a mother, she had done this FOUR TIMES – she knew what she was talking about. This woman was a goddess! She could have told me that the baby was going to come out of my big toe and I would have believed her! Chatting over coffee after the class with some of the other pregnant women, we all remarked at how lovely and knowledgeable Barbara was. She put us at ease and inspired confidence.

I spent about 7 years firmly believing that having your own children was essential to be a good, credible midwife. I started my midwifery programme when my older child was aged six. I was one of only seven, in a class of 25, who had children. This fact surprised me – still stubbornly believing that only mothers make good midwives.

The tide started to turn when I was nearing the end of my first year of midwifery training. By now I'd had some experience and exposure to caring for pregnant and labouring women and to several midwives' ways of practising. I saw some wonderful, caring midwives being so supportive and treating women as individuals. However, I also started to see that some of the midwives I was working alongside seemed unkind and uncaring; they sometimes imposed their personal labour experiences on women in a negative way. For example:

> Your baby is back to back, that's why your labour is taking so long. My labour was exactly the same, I took the epidural, you should really think about doing the same, you've got a long way to go yet.

This took me by surprise. I had seen other midwives in similar scenarios being similarly honest with women about why labour was taking a long time, but without attaching personal experiences or negativity. Instead they'd suggested ways of helping to turn the baby and coping with the hours ahead.

Some of my fellow mother midwifery students also expressed disgust about breastfeeding. I was shocked and wondered how they would support a woman postnatally at her lowest point, exhausted, in the middle of the night and looking for help to latch her baby for the umpteenth time. I also saw midwives who simply did not seem to care or have patience to provide care for women. This may have been because, as Flint (1989) suggests, childless midwives treat women unkindly because they are fostering issues of unresolved grief for their own childlessness. My experience of witnessing such treatment was not unique to the childless midwives though. For the first time I started to realise that some midwives who were mothers were actually not that supportive in a way that I would like to be supported. At the same time I realised that there were some fabulous midwives out there who had not yet become mothers themselves.

Could this really be true? You don't have to be a mother to be a good midwife? There is little written on this topic in academic journals in recent years. Therefore, I decided to look to the internet as one of my sources of information to gauge current public and professional opinion on this topic. Amongst the midwives who discussed this on a midwifery internet forum (Midwifery Sanctuary 2013) the consensus was that having children certainly was not a prerequisite to being a good midwife. Some, in fact, felt it had a negative impact:

> I think that my childbearing experience has had a detrimental effect on my practice . . .

Some childless midwives admitted that they felt obliged to lie to women who asked them if they had their own children. This was due to fear of the woman losing trust in her if she admitted she had not experienced childbirth.

> I squirm every time a woman asks me if I have children and I can see some of them droop visibly when I say 'No' – I realise some of them are asking out of interest but many are asking because they want to see that I know what I'm talking about.

However, those questioned who had had children after becoming midwives felt that their journey into motherhood had enhanced their skills. This supports Bewley's (2000b) finding that midwives acknowledged that their childbearing experience was life-changing and could actually enhance practice:

> Before I had my own child I didn't think it made any difference at all. However, since having a baby of my own I do think it has changed the way I feel about my job and how I respond to women, and I have become a better midwife because of it.

I think I was a good empathetic midwife before, but experience developed some aspects of my insight.

This leads us to the issue of the type of childbirth experience one has been through. Yes, I have had three children. I have been through spontaneous labour three times and have birthed my children vaginally. However, I have never had labour induced, experienced an epidural, a caesarean, or forceps – or any of hundreds of different scenarios that we deal with in our midwifery practice.

> I have children but I have never been in labour, women don't ask about that do they?

They just ask 'do you have any children?' I reply just 'yes' and then they often do seem to relax a little.

This suggests that it is too simplistic to segregate those with and those without children. There are myriad different types of childbirth experience and reasons why midwives are childless. It may be through choice, pregnancy loss, death or even gender. Male midwives are few in number, but one confirmed that he was asked if he had children; it was, however, in connection with competence with babies and not an expectation of shared reproductive experience (Bewley 2000b). Another who shared his thoughts on The Midwifery Sanctuary said that a fairly small percentage of women asked him if he had children – around 10 per cent. He was asked more by the partners of the women he cared for. This might imply that the question is an exercise in social bonding between men.

So when a woman asks me 'do you have children yourself' is she really saying 'do you know what I'm going through here?' I always answer honestly that I have given birth three times. I am, however, deliberately vague about the types of births I have had, instead emphasising that every pregnancy, labour and birth is very different.

Some childless midwives suggested that women for whom they cared were similarly reassured by length of experience as opposed to whether or not they had children:

> The odd time if they say 'How do you know?!' when I say 'I know' when they are saying how much it hurts etc, I reply that I have seen lots of women go through it . . . and how happy they were at the end. I think now I can say I've been qualified 'X' number of years, it makes me and them feel better, regardless of the children factor.

> I can honestly say I've never really perceived any 'issue' when I say no (when questioned about having children), and I too can back up my comments with midwifery experience these days which I agree women find reassuring.

Perhaps we should consider perceptions of what does make a good midwife and does that mean different things to different women in different situations? The midwives questioned in Rowan's (2003) qualitative study exploring the feelings and experiences of childless midwives study felt that care, sensitivity and competence were preferable to personal experience of childbirth. Are women equating age and life experience with midwifery experience? This is a simple enough assumption to make given that in the twentieth century people became midwives in their early twenties and stayed in until retirement. So older midwives had invariably had many years of midwifery experience. Nowadays, those entering midwifery do so at various stages of their lives, sometimes after their families are complete and grown up.

Turning to what the women think about this topic, there were extensive discussion threads on an internet parenting forum (Mumsnet 2013), which included some strong opinions on both sides:

> I have more respect for advice given to me by women with children, than those without.

> Motherhood is something you HAVE to experience to give accurate advice in my opinion.

I think childless midwives/health visitors can be good at their jobs, but they can't REALLY understand what it's like to be pregnant/give birth/breastfeed/ deal with more than one child etc . . . until they have actually experienced it.

I think it might often depend more on the person than whether they have their own children or not.

Making ill thought-out assumptions and judgements is not the preserve of the childless.

Sometimes a professional who has had children is worse because they make assumptions about themselves and about you/your family!

Yet people I know (medical and otherwise) who don't have kids can provide really useful advice because they are good at listening, identifying the main issue, questioning, guiding and empathy.

I think it's more that some people are more skilled than others than that motherhood is an essential additional experience.

A clear running theme was that the majority of contributors had asked their midwives if they had had children. So clearly women attach some importance to this information, as recognised by midwives (Bewley 2000a, 2000b; Rowan 2003).

It is interesting to note the changes over the last 60 years or so in both the socio-economic and demographic groups to which those working as midwives belong. Popular recent television serials have perfectly demonstrated this. *Call the Midwife* (BBC Television), although a dramatisation, is based on the memoirs (Worth 2002) of a midwife working in post WWII docklands London. Many of the midwives featured were nuns. However, those who were not were mainly from middle-class families, single and childless, as was the norm in early twentieth-century pre-NHS Britain. This was probably due to entry to midwifery being restricted to those who could afford the training (Leap & Hunter 1993).

Childbearing women did not appear to place such great importance on whether their midwives had children as certainly it was the norm that they didn't. Bewley (2000b) found when conducting her research that there are no current data available on the actual number of midwives with children. It may be reasonable, however, to assume that given changes in demographics, a greater percentage of women who now enter midwifery will have their own children. Has this then influenced what women now expect of their midwives?

In contrast, *One Born Every Minute* (Channel 4) portrays a fly-on-the-wall style documentary of a busy North of England maternity unit. It could be said that this unit is a reasonably accurate reflection of many large maternity units in the UK. Midwives featured in this programme come from a variety of backgrounds, including many who describe their own childbearing experiences on air. Although it was 1993 when Leap and Hunter considered midwifery to be open to women of all social classes and backgrounds, the same is true today.

An increasingly litigious culture and rapid technological progress means that great faith is now placed in the medical profession being able to 'fix anything'. With this assumption comes a greater emphasis on the skill of the midwife being able to produce a 'perfect outcome'. Women have lost faith in their own bodies and the natural process of birth which may contribute to women seeking reassurance about the midwife's skills and abilities.

I don't think any of us can say that we are the perfect midwife for every woman because each of us has our own philosophy of midwifery care, and each woman has her own expectations of her childbearing experience and different emotional and physical needs. My own observations of what I feel are unkind or unsupportive midwifery care are based on my own expectations of how I would like to be cared for. Thus the best we can do is try to treat each woman as an individual, listen to her needs, support her wishes and be competent and thoughtful. None of these carries the prerequisite of being a mother.

References

Bewley, C. (2000a) 'Personal experiences and midwifery practice: midwives without children', in M. Kirkham (ed.) *The Midwife-Mother Relationship*. Macmillan: Basingstoke: 169–92.

Bewley, C. (2000b) 'Feelings and experiences of midwives without children caring for childbearing women'. *Midwifery* 16: 135–44.

Flint, C. (1989) *Sensitive Midwifery*. London: Heinemann.

Leap, N. and Hunter, B. (1993) *The Midwife's Tale*. London: Scarlet Press.

Mander, R. (2009) 'The midwife who is not a mother', in R. Mander and V. Fleming (eds) *Becoming a Midwife*. London: Routledge.

Rowan, C. (2003) 'Midwives without children'. *British Journal of Midwifery* 11: 1 28–33.

Worth, J. (2002) *Call the Midwife*. Twickenham: Merton Books.

Internet sources

Mumsnet. http://www.mumsnet.com/Talk/am_i_being_unreasonable/a1602098-To-think-people-without-children-can-have-a-view. Accessed February 2013.

Midwifery Sanctuary. http://studentmidwivessanctuary.com/index.php?sid=abc327ff072e31b6401a8ed16f77d2d6. Accessed January 2013.

One Born Every Minute (Channel 4). http://www.channel4.com/programmes/one-born-every-minute/4od. Accessed June 2013.

Commentary

Indeed 'do you have children?' is a question that seems to have been addressed to me by every woman for whom I have cared on every continent. As Carrie says, the answer carries weight with women who expect midwives who have given birth to have a better understanding of their experience. Yet this was not always the case. Neither in the Old Testament, nor in ancient Egypt where midwives are referred to, is it stated that they have to have experience of childbirth. Indeed in the times of the Roman Empire this is an exclusion criterion, with it coming into fashion in Europe in the middle ages.

During my own doctoral studies the matter rose again in one interview with the participant stating:

> a lot of women believe you have to have given birth to be a good midwife. I think it's special if you've got that as well, it can be, but it can also be quite damaging if you have a poor experience of giving birth. I actually know of a midwife who had a very bad birth experience and the way she relates to women in labour is, to me, not good at all.
>
> *(Fleming 1994, p. 157)*

The negative aspects are clearly seen in this extract and Carrie draws similar links. Carrie admits to 'doing a U-turn' regarding her own thoughts on the matter. She also highlights the issue of the experience of labour and birth the midwife may have had. For every woman this is different and she cautions against midwives projecting their own experiences upon the women in their care. Indeed, qualitative researchers recognise that every experience is individual and their published work seeks to present these individual voices and not to generalise in the manner of quantitative researchers. A well carried-out international qualitative study on this theme is waiting to be done. Surely it will yield rich results.

Reference

Fleming, V. (1994) 'Partnership, politics and power'. PhD thesis, Massey University, New Zealand.

13

THE MIDWIFE WHO IS AN AUTHOR

Penny Curtis

VIGNETTE

Some years ago now, I was responsible for drafting an article for publication in an academic journal. I had been involved, with a colleague, in the evaluation of a small-scale pilot project to establish a practice initiative. Colleagues responsible for procuring funding, planning, and establishing and running the project were highly committed both professionally and emotionally to its success. That we could demonstrate that the project worked was, not surprisingly, important to them and they were concerned to do their best for all involved. My co-researcher and I were brought in, in the final few months of the project, when we planned and executed a realistic evaluation, reported the findings and eventually began the process of writing up elements for publication and dissemination to a broader professional and academic audience.

The article that I drafted explored the concept of empowerment and the facilitators and barriers to empowerment within the practice setting. One of the key themes that we wished to consider was the extent to which the realities of practice may lead to divergence in the nature of the involvement of members of different groups. Our evaluation suggested that the project's overarching aims and objectives became less central to the activities of some participants as new opportunities developed for them over time.

We felt that this was an important message and that acknowledgement and discussion of the potential for such 'organic' change was of value within midwifery, suggesting as it did that what comes to matter about an initiative –

the outcomes that people work towards – may not always be wholly predictable at the outset. Where such different outcomes become important, they have the potential to influence, positively or negatively, what happens in practice.

While some members of the project team shared our belief that this was a worthwhile issue to discuss in the academic and professional literature, we also encountered considerable opposition. We were asked to consider the implications of reporting such a finding for future funding: if we were suggesting that different parties were working to advance different objectives, would this not invalidate or at least undermine the initiative as a whole? Was there a danger that our paper might undermine the confidence of the funder in the project outcomes? We were also asked to take particular care in acknowledging the limitations of the evaluation process: concern for client confidentiality meant that the service initiative had been set up in a way that made it difficult to access a key group of participants in the evaluation, or to collect a form of data that we felt would have extended its analytical potential.

Discussion did not resolve these issues and we were unable to reconcile differences between interested parties. We could not find a way to write this article which did not provoke conflict with and within the project team: in the end, we did not submit the article for publication.

This experience raises two fundamental, though related, questions; first, why should the midwife author, and, second, are there circumstances in which midwives have a moral and/or ethical responsibility to write? I will reflect upon my own experience as I return to these questions, but first it is important to locate the midwife-as-author and ask who writes and in what contexts?

Who is the midwife author?

The midwife author may wear a variety of hats, sometimes successively, sometimes interchangeably. The student entering the midwifery profession may have much to say about the process of socialisation as they encounter and become immersed in the world of midwifery practice. Their educational experience may cause them to reflect upon or synthesise knowledge in a new way that has the potential to inform others in the profession or spark debate. Once in practice, midwives confront, on a daily basis, case study material, deficits in the existing knowledge base, ethical dilemmas and ongoing research and professional development issues which may all prompt the practising midwife to write. Managers, confronting the rapid pace of health service change and the barrage of difficulties that they encounter in attempting to deliver a quality service, may write in an effort to influence the political environment as they witness the pressures upon colleagues responsible for the provision of direct client care. Authorship may be fuelled by a desire to improve practitioners' working conditions and the birth experiences of childbearing women, or to demonstrate the benefits of practice initiatives that managers have introduced and supported. The research midwife may be obliged to publicise research methods and findings from research studies: to demonstrate benefit; to discuss lack of effect; to fulfil the requirements of funders; and to bolster employers' research outputs. Authorship may therefore be differently intentioned, and any and all of these differently positioned midwives may write with an eye to career development or career change.

Perhaps uniquely, however, the midwife academic has little option but to write. Writing for publication is a core aspect of an academic role and one that many of us struggle with to a greater or lesser extent. It is from my own standpoint of authoring as part of an academic role that I continue this discussion. Though there will inevitably be differences between my own perspectives and experiences and those of colleagues authoring in other roles, I hope that there will also be issues and experiences that resonate across roles.

A standpoint view – why should midwives author?

I concluded the vignette of one of my own authoring experiences by asking why should the midwife author? To consider this question I want to think about writing both as a process and as an outcome. By process, I refer to the 'doing' of writing: the undertaking of the task. Outcome refers to the finished project and the experiences that may be associated with having accomplished – and published – a piece of authored work.

The writing process can constitute an important developmental learning experience in its own right. Working through a writing task from conception of an idea, through planning, to crafting, editing and completion requires the author to demonstrate learning and a range of critical skills; not the least of these are organisation, synthesis and critique. The process of authoring requires every writer to clarify their thinking and develop their ability as a communicator.

There are, of course, inevitably challenges and pitfalls waiting in store for the would-be midwife author. The writing process requires what is often a precious resource – time! And time to think, to plan and to execute the writing task rarely seems to be available in abundance. The benefits to the midwife of working through the process of authoring have, it always seems, to be carved out of an already over-committed day.

Yet when this is possible and space to write does become available, authorship can bring a tremendous sense of achievement. Finding out that your first piece of work has been accepted for publication is memorable: that is my work! I wrote that! Others felt that what I have to say is worth printing! Seeing a piece of written work that you have authored come out in print can give a tremendous buzz! But more than this, the midwife who is a published author assumes a public position with respect to ongoing debate and to knowledge generation. The published author has committed to an opinion; they have taken a stance and communicated a perspective on an issue. They have put down a marker which often forms an important element of individual assessment in institutional staff reviews and appraisals. Publication may also help to position the individual, in a professional and an academic context, within a hierarchy of prestige.

There is clearly, therefore, benefit for the midwife author both in terms of the process of writing and in the outcome. However, the potential benefits of authorship do not only operate at the individual, personal level, but extend to the broader midwifery community and the midwifery profession as a whole. For the midwife in an academic role, published outputs help to indicate and sustain a 'critical mass' of scholarship, evidencing a supportive research environment which may increase the success of future research funding and studentship applications as well as stimulating the recruitment of research students. The midwife's profile as a published author is protective of the academic department, helping to build professional presence and prestige. Increasingly, the quality of midwives' authorship – in common with colleagues in other areas of academia – is subject to formal processes of research quality assessment, as they are required to participate in sector-wide appraisal schemes that are beginning to emerge in a number of countries (Key Perspectives 2009).

Authoring in context

In the UK, what began as a national Research Assessment Exercise (RAE) has evolved into the Research Excellence Framework (REF), the application of which, from 2014, will have far-reaching implications, influencing the allocation of research funding, defining how we understand the benefits to broader society of research carried out in the Higher Education sector, providing 'benchmarking information' and establishing 'reputational yardsticks' (REF 2014). In the UK, therefore, research quality assessment has direct implications for the sustainability and financial well-being of academic departments in what is increasingly a (global) market-driven model of higher education.

But more than this, such formal mechanisms of research quality assessment have a number of other implications – real and potential – for all midwife authors. The UK's REF currently rates authors' publications on a 5-point scale from unclassified through to 4-star (for the 2014 return, outputs – predominantly publications – will contribute 65 per cent to the overall Excellence profile; 20 per cent will be associated with research impact; and 15 per cent to the research environment). Only research outputs deemed to be world leading (4★) or internationally excellent (3★) will factor into the financial and prestige returns for institutions: outputs that are recognised internationally (2★) or that are recognised nationally (1★) in terms of originality, significance and rigour are, by implication, of limited value. Given the financial significance of the REF returns to institutions, the impact that such high value thresholds will have on midwifery authorship, and particularly on those midwives who are early in their authoring careers, will only become clear over time.

With the development of formal research assessment strategies, there has also been an increasing tendency to formalise and impose a hierarchy of publication outputs: in midwifery, peer-reviewed journal articles are super-valued over other forms of publication such as book chapters, authored books, reports etc. In Australia, the Excellence in Research for Australia initiative developed a 4-point journal ranking system (ARC 2009) in which discipline-specific, A* ranked journals were deemed to be qualitatively better than those with lower rankings. While used for the Australian 2010 Excellence exercise, journal ranking was subsequently discontinued though other metrics that 'measure the performance and/or impact of scholarly journals' (JournalMetrics 2013:3) are used, as they are in the UK, to assess journal quality. There is, therefore, pressure on midwives, sometimes subtle, sometimes overt, to make decisions about appropriate outlets for their writing that are based on which journals are highly cited, rather than which journals might reach the most appropriate audience. There is a real risk that this increasing focus on journal metrics exacerbates the existing dominance of English-language publishing and that it widens the division between practice-oriented and academic journals. Will we see, in the future, a situation in which practice-based midwives' authoring is largely confined to a sub-set of 'lower prestige' journals while their academic, university-based colleagues focus increasingly on high status journals that sustain an insular process of colleague citation?

Do midwives have an ethical and/or moral responsibility to write?

Given the potential benefits of authorship, and some of the contemporary pressures on authors, we need therefore to also consider the circumstances in which a midwife might choose not to author, recognising that the exercise of this responsibility may, at times, be uncomfortable. What the midwife author has to say may be challenging to others. With my own, unsuccessful writing experience that was described in the vignette, there was a singular failure to benefit the broader midwifery profession. In the face of opposition from experienced, well-respected colleagues, I failed to complete the authoring process and did not submit the article I had drafted for publication. The opportunity to disseminate what I considered to be important messages about a practice innovation was not realised.

Reflecting on this experience led me to consider my own moral and/or ethical responsibility to write. My failure to complete the authoring process has crystallised into a strong belief that midwives do indeed have a moral and, often, an ethical responsibility to write and to publish. This may not always be an easy responsibility to exercise, yet as members of a professional group with responsibility for client care, the onus is on the midwife to foster dialogue and to enable reflexive consideration of all aspects of professional ethos and practice. Dialogue is not only good for midwifery, it is essential. The midwife author has the potential to extend the knowledge base for midwifery practice, to contribute to evidence-based care and, just as importantly, to strengthen theoretical understandings – for theory and practice must inform one another. Through authorship, the midwife may disseminate research findings to a variety of user audiences, justify and extend aspects of midwifery practice and challenge others. There should be no no-go areas: if we cannot write about it, discuss it, critique it, this probably means that we cannot justify it. A profession that fears to air or acknowledge its own limitations surely threatens to undermine its own foundations and the basis for its independent existence. There would appear to be clear echoes here of the sentiments expressed in the Francis Report (2013). The report, which evidenced widespread, substandard care provided in one UK NHS Trust, called for 'openness, transparency and candour throughout the system about matters of concern' (Francis Report, p.4). The midwife as author has, therefore, a moral and an ethical obligation to write; to open up to scrutiny and debate (both professional and public) accepted ways of understanding, assumptions and practices.

Some reflections on the practice of writing

Exercising this obligation to write need not, however, be a solitary experience; indeed collaborating with others in pursuit of a writing project – either by co-authoring and/or through informal peer reviewing – can help to hone not just contributors' individual writing skills, but also a range of important teamworking skills.

In some areas, including biomedical research and practice, in which research typically takes place in large teams, the number of co-authors can be very extensive. This is much less common in midwifery, but co-authoring is, nevertheless, widely practised. It is not uncommon for writers to begin their publishing career by co-authoring with a more experienced clinical or academic colleague. At any stage in an author's writing career, co-authoring can be a stimulating process that allows all involved to realise writing projects that might otherwise be unattainable. In my experience, as a general principle, it is wise to know your co-author/s before embarking on a joint writing project. How do they think? What is it about the writing project that excites and drives them? How do they feel about the subject matter? From such understanding, trust may develop that allows for clear agreement about each contributor's input (particularly, its nature and timing) and the give and take necessary for co-authorship to take place to the benefit of all. Collaborative writing can provide support for the new writer, building confidence for the future and can sustain and energise the efforts of more experienced authors. Co-authoring can therefore be a stimulating and enjoyable process, whether practised with close peers or colleagues from broader professional and academic networks. In the academic context, this may entail collaboration with colleagues from other disciplines, other universities and even internationally.

Similar benefits may be available to the midwife author through the process of informal peer reviewing. Checking with others that what you wish to say is worth saying, and that the way that you are saying it is clear, is both worthwhile and a common practice for many authors, from the novice through to the experienced writer. Colleagues may lend important insights and constructive criticism in relation to your work. And this process need not, of course, be confined to midwifery colleagues.

Participating in writing as a collaborative process can therefore be very rewarding and has much to offer the midwife author, but it is not a universal panacea. At the heart of any collaborative venture author is a relationship between (usually busy) individuals and, like any relationship, it doesn't always work out and the result can be a messy and sometimes acrimonious divorce. Here, I am mindful of a much more recent, failed writing experience, which began when I committed to authoring a chapter in an edited book. I duly provided a short draft of the chapter's content for the editors. When the volume was commissioned, the requirements for my chapter had been amended to ensure coherence between all the contributing chapters. While this is not in itself unusual, unfortunately much of the amended content was outside of my experience – and more worryingly, outside of my area of interest – and a co-author had been appended. Although the nominated co-author was an experienced academic, for whom I had considerable respect, we had no prior experience of working together and no insights into each other's approach to, or perspective on, the issues to be discussed. We were unable to negotiate a shared vision for the writing project or to reconcile our expectations for the chapter. On this occasion, co-authoring did not work out and several months later, when offered the opportunity to withdraw from the authoring project I jumped at the chance, breathing a huge sigh of relief. While I recount this experience to insert a note of caution and to illustrate the potential pitfalls of attempting to write collaboratively, I have only once had such a negative experience in my own writing career and the positive, productive experiences have therefore far outweighed the negatives.

Getting words down on paper

Although the curriculum in English schools currently emphasises the different writing styles that are required for different forms of written communication, I suspect that many of us have reached adulthood with limited preparation for authoring. On the whole, no one teaches us how to write and authorship can invoke an uncomfortable feeling of insecurity. Mastering academic writing, in particular, may seem like mastering a foreign language; any midwife academic will readily describe the tendency for students to obscure what they are trying to say through the use of (what the student deems to be) 'academic' vocabulary. What, for example, did this doctoral student really mean to convey when they wrote, 'Always visible, breasts signify the transition from girlhood to womanhood they appear at a time when an identity of one-self is being formed and that identity is shaped by others perceptions of how our breasts match the ideal although not the normal, they are objects fixed on by a subject.'? Writing that does not communicate clearly leaves the reader with a lot of work to do to try to understand the meaning that the author intends to convey.

There are always, of course, colleagues who write fluidly, cogently and apparently spontaneously. To those of us who are less fortunate, the practice of writing can perhaps more accurately be described as 'like pulling teeth'. Writing, as the American novelist Paul Theroux is reputed to have said, 'is pretty crummy on the nerves' (Storyteller 2006).

There is a wealth of advice available to the budding author in books, on-line resources and writing for publication courses. These provide advice and suggest techniques for organising, writing and editing the writing project and some suggestions for further reading are included at the end of this chapter. Although there is no intention to summarise the available advice here, some aspects of the practice of writing are worth commenting upon – though in doing so I acknowledge that these are firmly embedded in my own experiences and other authors may well generate a very different emphasis.

There may only be a subtle distinction, at times, between 'drafting' and 'writing', but approaching a writing task as a draft can liberate the author to think about *what* they want to say rather than just *how* they want to say it.

Organisation is key: authoring often requires reorganisation, editing, further reorganisation, further editing . . . And so on.

It is at least as important for an author to decide what to keep out of their writing project as it is to decide what to put in.

If you get lost, and find yourself easily distracted from your writing task, look carefully at your organisation. Are you clear about what you are trying to say?

If you are really getting nowhere and feel as though you are going round in circles, take a break and come back with fresh eyes in a few hours or days or even weeks.

Never underestimate the importance of proofreading your work. Minor errors can radically change your meaning: 'aseptic technique' is but one press of a space bar away from 'a septic technique'.

Once you feel that you have completed the writing task, try to allow yourself time to set your work aside for a while so that you can come back to it with fresh eyes after a week or two. If there appear to be no glaring mistakes, issues or inconsistencies, then you may be ready to send it off for review.

Finally, if a particular piece of advice/technique does not work *for you*, do not be afraid to discard it and try something else. For example, it is sometimes suggested that a writer should commit to producing a set number of words per day, every day. This has never worked for me, though I know other authors who do use this approach.

In my own authorship, I struggle with organisation and am easily sidetracked. I have spent, over the years, what must amount to several days looking through the thesaurus for a precise word in order to craft a sentence. Eventually, I have come to accept that this is nothing more than a distraction, taking me away from the task of writing. However, even with acceptance, I still find myself doing this on occasions. For example, while writing this chapter I chose to look up the meaning of the word 'process' in on-line dictionaries. Process is a word that I use frequently and have little difficulty with. I did come across a new word –

'obviousism', which I am informed means 'an expression of obviousness' (Merriam-Webster 2013), but this has been of little use to me other than to illustrate how easy it is to distract myself from the task of writing! There is, of course, a plethora of opportunities for distraction. Perhaps even more problematic is my urge to find just one more paper before I start writing. Databases such as Google scholar just make it too easy to perpetuate the belief that an additional source will justify my arguments and raise my writing to a new level when, in reality, it serves only to delay the writing process itself.

The majority of authors probably have their own foibles. What matters is that where the midwife occupies a role that requires authorship, there is a need to reflect upon the challenges experienced and explore ways of managing these.

Some reflections on the process of getting published

As I have argued, some midwives, and particularly those working in the higher education sector, are subject to persistent and increasing pressure to publish. The moral and ethical issues that I perceived in relation to my own failure to publish were, in reality, only part of the picture: I also feared the loss of a publication opportunity. This pressure is, therefore, increasingly influenced by institutional considerations rather than the needs of practitioners or of the broader user community. The academic midwife has to balance a responsibility to practice colleagues and to childbearing women and their families with the increasing pressure, evident within the higher education (HE) sector, to target publications in light of externally defined quality criteria. Midwives working outside of the HE sector may experience different pressures upon them to prioritise particular forms of dissemination and publication. Ideally, however, decisions about how to craft a writing project, who the target audience should be, and what the best publication outlet is, should be made only after carefully considering a range of questions, some of which are highlighted below.

Have you got something new/different to say? Who do you want to read your work? Why should they? Where might you publish to make your work available to them? What is the most appropriate format? Do you know enough about your proposed publication medium? (for example, the aims and target audience of a journal). What sort of balance between academic/accessible language will best suit your target audience? – is this compatible with your intended publication medium? Can you write enough words for the medium (e.g. the journal article) that you have in mind? Or: can you say what you need to within the word constraints? Do you need your publication to carry with it other 'values'? (For example, does it need to be a peer-reviewed article? Does it need to be in a journal which ranks highly in the Citation Index?) Will your message still be current by the time others get to see it? (for example, by the time it gets through the publication cycle).

Although by no means exhaustive, these are suggestive of some of the questions an author might consider as they commit to a writing project and work towards getting published. The way in which an individual responds to these will vary over time and between projects; however, there are some considerations to be mindful of: Writing for different audiences often requires different presentational styles. Journals that concentrate on the audience that you intend to target will have a 'house style' which they deem to be effective as a means of communicating with their readership. The potential author may only get a feel for this style by identifying and carefully reading articles which have some similarity to the article under preparation. Familiarisation with this house style is different to, though no less important than, a thorough understanding of the guidance to authors which all journals provide. The latter clarifies key presentational elements expected for all submissions and should not be ignored. If a prospective author is unclear about whether a specific journal is an appropriate outlet for a writing project, having read the journal's aims and reviewed some of the articles already published, an enquiry directed at the editor is often possible. Once you are clear that you have targeted an appropriate outlet, submission is now usually achieved by means of what can seem to be a daunting, on-line submission system. From this point, several weeks of waiting can be expected, which may stretch into months for the more prestigious journals, before authors receive feedback on their submission.

One of the key techniques for quality assurance in the publication process is the use of anonymous refereeing of submitted articles. This means that the writing project that you submit will be independently reviewed – often by two members of an editorial board who have expertise in the subject area. These reviewers will make recommendations to the editor about the quality of your submission and its suitability for publication. For some, the process ends at this point with rejection by the journal. Having an article accepted for publication without the require-ment to undertake amendments is a very rare, perhaps mythical, experience. More frequently, authors receive anonymous (and even, sometimes, contradictory) comments from the reviewers and an invitation to re-submit a revised paper. This can be a challenging time for authors and the idea of undertaking substantial work on a writing project that had been completed and 'ticked off', can seem overwhelming. After the initial, perhaps inevitable disappointment and the benefit of reflection, reviewers' comments are usually insightful, constructive and aimed at improving – rather than destroying – the piece of work. However, it is important to recognise first, that the author does *not* have to agree with the reviewers' recommendations for change and, second, that amending an article in a manner that takes into consideration the comments of the reviewers does *not* guarantee that it will subsequently be accepted for publication.

For authors who successfully negotiate the publication process and whose articles are accepted by a journal, further delays are then encountered as the paper goes through the process of being formatted and prepared for print. After a long period of inactivity, a final effort is required from the author who must confirm the accuracy of the formatted paper before it goes into the journal's queue for publication. On-line journals and those that have on-line availability in advance of a printed copy may only have a short delay before the author can access their published output. However, a hard copy may still be many months away. The length of the publication cycle varies considerably between journals but it is often a long and a slow process. As Ann Thomson (2005 p.190) has noted 'Acceptance of a paper for publication sometimes appears to be a mountain that has to be climbed'. Importantly, however, if you stumble in the foothills and receive an initial rejection, don't give up! Take time to look critically at your article and if you are still convinced that you are saying something worthwhile, resubmit to a different outlet. One recent article that I am particularly fond of was submitted to three different journals before it was eventually published.

Summary

Authoring is fundamental to the credibility and development of the midwifery profession. Differently positioned midwives may experience authorship as a moral and ethical responsibility to varying degrees. A common factor, though, in the experience of many is a lack of proactive support to enable the ongoing development of confidence as a writer, and skill as a communicator through the medium of the written word.

For the midwife to author effectively they must know what they want to say, why it is worth saying and how it relates to the existing knowledge base. Though authoring can be highly pressured, and is not without its challenges, it can also be highly rewarding and an aspect of midwifery practice that we ignore at our peril.

Advice about writing

Books

Day, R.A. and Gastel, B. (2012) *How to Write and Publish a Scientific Paper*, 7th edition. Cambridge: Cambridge University Press.
Holland, K. and Watson, R. (eds) (2012) *Writing for Publication in Nursing and Healthcare: Getting it Right*. Oxford: Wiley-Blackwell.
Oermann, M.H. and Hays, J.C. (2010) *Writing for Publication in Nursing*, 2nd edition. Springer Publishing Company.
Rocco, T.S. and Hatcher, T. (eds) (2011) *The Handbook of Scholarly Writing and Publishing*. San Francisco, CA: John Wiley.

Journal articles: these include guidance and/or discussion about the writing and the publication process

A series of 12 accessible articles on writing for professional publication was authored by Dr John Fowler and published in the *British Journal of Nursing* between September 2010 and April 2011. The series considers the following issues: finding the motivation to write; defining your subject matter; following journal guidelines; supporting your statements; creating interest; writing the abstract; structure and presentation; targeting the right journal; using client case studies; publishing a project report; and writing conference abstracts.

Fahy, K. (2010) 'How to get published in an international journal' (editorial). *Women and Birth* 23(2): 43–4.

Happell, B. (2011) 'Responding to reviewers' comments as part of writing for publication'. *Nurse Researcher* 18(4): 23–7.

Marchant, S. (2010) 'Rigour and respect: Aspects for consideration when undertaking and publishing research'. *Midwifery* 26(3): 264–7.

Thomson, A.M. (2005) 'Writing for publication in this refereed journal'. *Midwifery* 21(2): 190–4.

References

ARC (2009) Tiers for the Australian Ranking of Journals http://www.arc.gov.au/era/tiers_ranking.htm. Accessed 5 April 2013.

Francis Report (2013) The Mid Staffordshire NHS Foundation Trust Public Inquiry – Chaired by Robert Francis QC. http://www.midstaffspublicinquiry.com/report. Accessed 30 May 2013.

JournalMetrics (2013) 'Frequently asked questions'. http://www.journalmetrics.com/FAQs.pdf (page 3). Accessed 5 April 2013.

Key Perspectives (2009) *A Comparative Review of Research Assessment Regimes in Five Countries and the Role of Libraries in the Research Assessment Process*. Report commissioned by OCLC Research. http://www.oclc.org/research/publications/library/2009/2009-09.pdf. Accessed 4 April 2013.

Merriam-Webster (2013) 'New words and slang'. http://nws.merriam-webster.com/opendictionary/newword_display_alpha.php?letter=Ob&last=50 (noun)

REF 2014. *The Research Excellence Framework*. http://www.ref.ac.uk/. Accessed 4 April 2013.

Storyteller (2006) 'Writing quotes'. http://www.writing.com/main/view_item/item_id/1066921-Writing-Quotes. Accessed 29 May 2013.

Thomson, A.M. (2005) 'Writing for publication in this refereed journal'. *Midwifery* 21(2): 190–94.

Commentary

Thankfully Penny's experience with writing the research report outlined in her vignette has not put her off completing this chapter, which takes the reader through a number of scenarios, not all of which are negative! Indeed Penny has an impressive track record of publication which shows that persistence pays off! She highlights important issues for the would-be midwife author. Because of the increasing competition amongst universities for funding, there is more and more pressure to publish in the highly ranked journals. Possibly this has led not only to research findings reaching the wrong audience, as Penny has explained, but also to an increasing number of rejections for individual writers. In turn, this is time consuming and frustrating as the value of carefully planned, executed and important work appears to be challenged by reviewers. Penny has proposed one way to help overcome this: writing with a more experienced colleague. This is a very valuable suggestion but it is not always a guarantee of success. Writing for peer-reviewed journals therefore requires a thick skin and, as is highlighted here, a willingness to be flexible and change or even remove what may seem to be key parts of the text to comply with reviewers' requests. Penny's final piece of advice is something all intending authors must hold dear i.e. know what to say, why it is worth saying and how it builds on what is already known.

14

ON NOT BECOMING A MIDWIFE

The role of the birth activist

Nadine Edwards

When Rosemary Mander first invited me to write this chapter, my thoughts immediately went to an *Association for Improvements in the Maternity Services* (AIMS) *Journal* article written by Nancy Stewart, a remarkable birth activist, erstwhile *AIMS Journal* editor, and 'thwarted midwife'. I searched through each *AIMS Journal* backwards and was about to give up, when I finally spotted it in the Autumn 1983 edition. There it was: 'Confessions of a thwarted midwife' (Stewart 1983). It is a piece that stayed with me since I first read it all those years ago, because it resonated deeply with how I felt. Lynn Walcott's (2009) article from *Midwifery Matters, Journal for the Association of Radical Midwives* (ARM) could have been written as its sequel, and was equally resonating. It also seemed somehow fitting to begin with AIMS and ARM, given their radical roots and affiliations.

VIGNETTE

Throughout Britain there is a small but growing number of frustrated women. . . . These women – and I am one – are thwarted midwives. These are women who have children of their own. And who through their own experiences of pregnancy, birth and motherhood feel drawn to support and love other women and families. Generally, they have involved themselves in the periphery of birth, through various voluntary organisations. But what they feel is a calling to do more than that . . . As midwifery selection and training is currently organised in this country, there is little chance that these thwarted midwives and the health system will come together. And the rejection, unhappily, is often mutual. . . . It

---

would seem that the direct entry course, a 3-year programme without prior nursing training, would be especially appropriate for pulling in experienced women who know they want to be midwives (*not* nurses). But the NHS doesn't see it that way, or just doesn't value the experience of motherhood in its midwives. There are pitifully few direct entry courses available and they are difficult to enter.

(Stewart 1983:4)

Nancy went on to explain that the few direct entry places available were predominantly given to young women, and that woman with older children and women who had shown an interest in birth by working for voluntary organisations like AIMS were usually rejected:

They may shy away from a woman's prior knowledge, fearing that she wouldn't toe the line. Perhaps they're right. Because that's the other side of the incongruence between many 'natural midwives' and the existing structure. . . . They fear that they would not only not learn what they need to know, but also would learn attitudes and approaches that are inconsistent with the kind of midwives they want to be.

(Stewart 1983:8)

Nancy ended her short article by suggesting that parents should have the right to choose their birth attendants, and that 'thwarted midwives' could be:

invited labour helpers, who stay with a couple at home or in hospital, not replacing professional attendants but offering a service too often absent in birth today – the attentive support of a known and trusted companion throughout labour, who is not involved in hospital routines or hierarchies, but is centred totally on the needs of the labouring woman and her partner.

(Stewart 1983:8)

The current-day doula, in fact?

To become midwives, Nancy explained that 'thwarted midwives' would either have to compromise their ideals, or the training system would have to change to welcome them.

Although I was very much one of these 'thwarted midwives', and although I have attended births as a supportive presence since 1982, I have not trained to become a midwife. This is partly because while direct entry midwifery courses are now widely available, the underlying problems described by Nancy have not been entirely resolved. Other reasons are eloquently described in former independent midwife Lynn Walcott's (2009) article:

There were such sacrifices in the beginning to become a midwife. My story is a familiar one; married with children, I got the calling to become a midwife in my 20s. I spent years preparing to apply, waiting for the right time for me and my family . . . the training was about making me 'one of them' – I must fit in – it is the only way to survive . . . I felt woefully inadequate going into that first job.

(Walcott 2009:10)

On 'Delivery suite . . . already feeling the pressure of 'being different', resorting to 'hid[ing] in the bathroom with a Pinard', Lynn then moved to a private birth centre and then to an NHS community post, and 'Yes, I knew some of these women well, but I was still sharing the care – my caseload was too big to give complete one-to-one care' (Walcott 2009:10–11).

Finally becoming an independent midwife (see chapter 10), Lynn described this as ideal for her, until recent years, when independent midwives have become increasingly 'managed' and under 'close tabs'. Lynn explained that this is due to a divergence in philosophy between NHS and independent midwifery, with the NHS philosophy increasingly encroaching on the practice of independent midwives:

I no longer feel 'independent'. I am checked, and measured, and followed, and questioned . . . my kind of midwifery is considered 'misconduct' . . . strike that midwife off who does not conform to the obstetric ideal! . . . In my heart I will always be a midwife – just not the registered kind, official, within the law, controlled, practising.

(Walcott 2009:12).

These two personal stories, perhaps more than any others express why I didn't, and have continued, not to become a midwife, despite a strong and consistent calling spanning over 30 years.

The beginnings of the calling to becoming a midwife

As we know and as is well documented, the 1970s saw the consolidation of a largely medicalised approach to birth. Birth technologies were not only increasing apace, but were being used routinely in the UK and in most high-income countries, with the exception of the Netherlands (Davis-Floyd *et al.* 2013). While the caesarean rate was still relatively low in high-income countries in the 1970s, the use of oxytocin for induction of labour, shaving of pubic hair and enemas at the start of labour, the use of pethidine for pain relief, syntometrine to expel the placenta, separation of mothers and babies at birth and the days after birth, long hospital stays, poor breastfeeding support and regimented routines for mothers and babies were prolific. At the same time, the so-called 'hippy' era had ignited undercurrents of unease and dissatisfaction with mainstream thinking, and our increasingly capitalist, technocratic, and mechanistic ways of thinking and living.

Becoming pregnant in this context, in my late teens, was, not surprisingly, a formative life experience. Naïve perhaps, and lacking in knowledge, I nonetheless had an innate and unshakeable belief in my body's ability to give birth without the need for the drugs and technologies available at the time. I had memories of my youngest sibling being born at home, and thought this was normal. Despite a dearth of information (the findings of the Birthplace study were light years away), I managed to find a copy of Frederick Leboyer's, *Birth Without Violence* (1975). I tracked down the Society to Support Home Confinements, founded by Margaret Whyte, and discovered Marjorie Tew's work on the safety of home birth (I am ever grateful to the friend who gave me Margaret's address and for the work Margaret did to keep home birth alive through the 1970s and 80s). I felt lionesquely protective towards my unborn baby, more informed, and was convinced that I could best avoid interventions that might hurt or damage my baby by staying at home. Relatively well armed, I was still unprepared for the injection of syntometrine that was unceremonioulsy jabbed into my thigh at birth, without so much as a by-your-leave – far less informed consent.

Interestingly, those of us in rural and semi-rural areas often met fierce opposition to birthing at home, but the alternative we were pressured to agree to was small cottage hospitals, where the facilities were very similar to those at home. All in all it was an awakening to the politics of birth, and the beginnings of a long journey.

Becoming a birth activist

Passionate about the implications of birth for women, babies and their families and three babies later, by some fortuitous coincidence, I was 'found' by AIMS and invited to join. In the days before Google and email, this was no mean feat, as AIMS was a small group with precious few members in Scotland. I never looked back. It quickly became my source of inspiration, knowledge and, above all, support. The AIMS Committee comprises, at any one time, one of the most thinking, caring and honest groups of women I know. Their continuing integrity is second to none. Yet in its early days, and even now, 'AIMS members have long been used to being cast as the strident, complaining voices of the minority . . . self-indulgent romantics caring more for a pleasant experience than the lives of ourselves and our babies' (Stewart 1989:3).

I was fortunate enough to train on the first Birth Teachers Course through the London Birth Centre, and started pregnancy groups in Edinburgh in 1985 (www.pregnancyandparents.org). While unsure about what I had to offer, I wanted to provide a safe place for women to share their knowledge and experiences, provide the information that I had been exposed to through AIMS, and (given the embodied nature of birth) I thought that breathing and yoga (called body work then) might be helpful. My small but growing library was central to these groups, with books by authors such as Sally Inch, Beverley Beech and Ina May Gaskin. My contact with pregnant women through AIMS, and my pregnancy groups led to me being asked by a few women to support them through their labours and births, nearly always at home. Most had had to show the 'patience of Job, the courage of Joan of Arc and the political skill of a Metternich' (Donnison 1988:195) in order to secure midwifery care for their home births and wanted support not to waver from their decision. In modern-day parlance, I was being asked to be an advocate and doula. Most gave birth at home as planned, but sometimes they felt unable to call midwives until late in labour, or felt that they had to keep them at a distance in some other way. Mostly midwives ignored me, or were occasionally hostile towards me, but I stayed quiet, offering support in the best way I could. It was this enormous privilege of being asked to be with women and their families through birth that awakened most strongly my calling to becoming a midwife. Initially, I wanted to be able to provide the kind of holistic midwifery care, built on a relationship of trust, that I had wanted during my own pregnancies and birth, and that the women who asked me to be at their births clearly wanted and needed. Going into labour in battle mode is less than ideal (as we now know only too well), and I felt increasingly frustrated that I could not offer midwifery care as well as friendship and support. I also wanted to add my voice to the voices of those courageous midwives who have and continue to advocate for women, babies and their families, who understand the pivotal role of the midwife in sustainable birthing practices and strengthening families and communities, especially those suffering from multiple and endemic disadvantages (Davies *et al.* 2011; Reed & Walton 2009).

Still feeling the sentiments expressed in Nancy's poignant piece on 'thwarted midwives' and still campaigning for a direct entry programme in Lothian, I continued to be involved in 'the periphery of birth' (Stewart 1983:4), though it didn't necessarily feel peripheral: running pregnancy and postnatal groups, attending births, reading research, writing for the *AIMS Journal*, providing phone, face-to-face and eventually email support and information, attending conferences, sitting on committees and being involved in an inspiring Edinburgh AIMS/ARM group. This group of four AIMS members and four ARM midwives taught me about the value of women and midwives working together, our commonalities and the importance of understanding each other's experiences, knowledge and points of view.

The beginnings of moving away from becoming a midwife

Just as direct entry courses were becoming more available, and my children were getting older, by another set of fortuitous coincidences, I was given the welcome, if unexpected, privilege of starting a PhD in 1994 at the University of Edinburgh. While completing this PhD on women's experiences of planning home births (Edwards 2005), it became very clear to me that for the reasons Nancy and Lynn wrote about, I could not train to become, or practise, as a midwife in the current climate.

Listening carefully to the women in my study explain about the untold harm that had been or could be inflicted upon them through the routine use of birth interventions and watching close colleagues train as midwives, striving to retain their integrity while being asked to carry out procedures they believed to be unnecessary and potentially harmful, consolidated my view. As Nancy's article described, I was one of those women who had to conclude (despite positive changes during the intervening years) that I still could not train as a midwife. While the sadness of an unfulfilled calling remains, there are many ways of working on the 'periphery' – many ways of working towards positive change.

Like the many 'thwarted midwives' described in Nancy's article, I continued to be a 'not quite midwife', by continuing to be a birth supporter – forerunner to the contemporary doula. Birth activists and midwives alike have turned to doula-ism, in order to offer emotional and practical support to women and families, to be able to build a trusting relationship with them, and to be able to focus on the woman rather than on the woman's notes and institutional requirements. Just as the birth activist before her, the doula has attracted much debate (Stockton 2012). Importantly, the doula has also been described as a response to the state of current maternity services – to be both an advocate and empathetic companion in a fragmented and technological environment – taking on the previous role of the midwife. Some even see this as a move towards the emergence of lay midwifery, as these women learn about birth and midwifery empirically and promote confidence in women's abilities to birth their babies.

Accepting the 'outsider' role

As I mentioned earlier, those of us working though organisations like AIMS, on what has been described as the 'outside', were often viewed with disdain or even open hostility. And while this persists in some quarters, generally there is a greater feeling of solidarity and acceptance that AIMS has a valuable role to play in improving maternity services and advocating for midwives as well as for women. Those of us working with AIMS value and appreciate those midwives who align themselves with women, who understand the importance of agency and support women to make their own decisions (especially those who have had few opportunities to do so), and who understand that birth is not just about having a baby, but about making a family and forming lifelong relationships. Likewise, midwives value and appreciate those outside midwifery who support them when they are criticised, even victimised, for what they do (AIMS 2011). Together we develop critiques for understanding the increasingly technological approach to birth, political tools for building initiatives to revolutionise birth practices and campaigns to protect and initiate social models of midwifery based on trusting relationships, respect and sharing of knowledge. This is our greatest strength and asset – this increasingly joint understanding that a social model of birth, supported by appropriate and timely technology when needed, in both high- and low-income countries, is both safe and sustainable for families, communities and the planet, and is best provided by skilled, culturally safe, midwives (with the caveat that we understand 'midwife' to mean all those with appropriate birth skills and knowledge and that this can be acquired through a variety of routes).

Translating women's voices into political activity

One of the useful aspects of remaining within activism is the potential to listen carefully to women's experiences and assimilate common threads and themes over time. AIMS is in the unique position of 'hearing it like it is', as AIMS President Jean Robinson rightly reminds us that we must. As former Chair of the Patients Association, in the 1970s Jean was one of the first to understand the damaging impact of routine induction on women, at a time when going against medical advice was described by one obstetrician as 'foolhardy' (Squire 1984:3). This vocal obstetrician claimed that: '"extremist" groups are urging mothers-to-be to refuse procedures such as induction, foetal heart monitoring and caesarean section' (Squire 1984:3). AIMS has often been called to account for holding a dangerously radical position and yet, again and again, subsequent research has proved it right to raise the concerns it has. Women's experiences can act as an early warning system, as in the distressing case of women being awake during caesareans under general anaesthetic. It was the voices of these women that led AIMS Chair Beverley Beech to the shocking realisation that not only was this happening, but that these women were disbelieved (Beech 1985). Better known campaigns have included getting fathers into the birth room, getting rid of routine shaving and enemas in early labour, reducing episiotomy rates, reducing the routine use of drugs to expel the placenta, raising awareness about the potential harms of routine ultrasound (particularly its commercial use) and promoting birth in the community. Another important campaign focused on increasing normal birth rates. Research was subsequently carried out on the numbers of normal births and the Royal College of Midwives launched its own Normal Birth campaign. A recent campaign, A Midwife for Me, brings together a range of midwifery and lay organisations (AIMS, NCT, ARM, Independent Midwives UK, The Birth I Want and Birthrights) to press for caseloading midwifery, with built-in incentives for midwives who want to provide this kind of care (M4M 2013).

Yet, as far back as 1991, an AIMS editorial suggested that the 'work of AIMS sometimes seems like the efforts of a flea, nibbling the hindquarters of a charging bull in an attempt to change his direction' (Stewart 1991:1). While turning the juggernaut around still feels nigh impossible, AIMS and other organisations and activists continue to represent women's experiences and challenge outmoded beliefs and practices through Maternity Services Liaison Committees (MSLCs), assisting in the development of NICE Guidelines and Cochrane Reviews, lobbying government officials, contributing to government reports on maternity services and more. Indeed, the role of the birth activist is to challenge – carefully and thought- fully – for, as Mary Nolan suggested, 'challenge is the life blood of improvement' (2011:17).

The right to represent?

But on what basis does an organisation like AIMS represent women's views? When a message is unpalatable, the messenger often bears the brunt, and AIMS has frequently been accused of representing a small number of disgruntled middle-class women. The issue of representation has long been debated, and Charlotte Williamson's (1992) writings clarified this debate. She explained how providers and recipients of health care form different and valuable perspectives and advocated for the informed lay perspective, based on years of listening to many voices. Her argument is not dissimilar to the standpoint of theorists and feminists, the essence of which suggests that those on the receiving end of mainstream thinking and practices have different and often more piercing insights than those who perpetuate these unquestioningly. The rich tapestry of experience from those on the receiving end is exactly what AIMS can bring. Yet, dislike of a knowledgeable voice remains, in some quarters:

> as lay people become more knowledgeable and develop more understanding of the professions, health services and clinical issues, they lose their amateur status and, thus, their value. Like the wise fool of mythology lay people's innocence and naiveté are considered useful by professionals, managers and health service commentators. Knowledgeable individuals are considered unrepresentative of other lay people. In particular, activist members of voluntary lay groups are liable to be regarded as unrepresentative (atypical) and, therefore, unable to represent (voice) the views of their peers.
>
> *(Hogg and Williamson 2001:4)*

In researching women's experiences of being on MSLCs, this is exactly what I sometimes found. This was aptly captured by one woman describing her experience:

> I realised I kind of turned up and I had my birth experiences and I shared those and was told, well anecdotes – not helpful and the research says blah. So I cottoned on to the fact that research might be a helpful thing to be able to access . . . Once I kind of cracked that then it turned out I wasn't the right kind of user because I wasn't representative of the women using the service, as they wouldn't be able access that or interact in the MSLC. So anybody who can interact on the MSLC isn't actually very helpful because they're not representative of the women using the service.
>
> *(Nadine Edwards, unpublished interviews)*

The way forward

So much can be done on the 'periphery' described by Nancy, and yet, by not enabling both 'thwarted midwives' and midwives to contribute to positive change, the plight of midwifery remains. Nancy saw direct entry midwifery programmes, which would welcome women with families and embrace their knowledge, as a way of solving the 'thwarted midwife' problem, and to some extent this has happened. But Lynn's article, along with others, captures how challenging the midwifery training can be for those women, and that once qualified, there are few options for them to practice in ways they believe in – offering the possibility of trusting relationships, and providing respect and support for women's decisions when these fall outside usual guidelines and practice. Without the mutually trusting relationships central to Nancy's and Lynn's articles, neither mothers nor midwives can be the best mothers and midwives that they want to be. The deconstruction, destruction and privatisation of the NHS further serves to fragment and undermine relationships.

Additionally, the current rule-bound, fear-based trajectory towards standardisation of training, practice (and life in general) is constraining rather than innovative (Kirkham 2013). Coupled with decreasing resources in health and education, neither midwifery training nor practice can easily be embracing and creative. Many of the midwifery initiatives promoting the kind of practices Lynn described, which lead to good outcomes and high levels of satisfaction for women and midwives, have been dismantled or are under threat: The Albany Midwifery Practice has gone, and independent midwifery as we know it, is on the brink of extinction.

One question raised by Nancy and Lynn concerns whether we could and should change the increasingly homogenous midwifery education and practice. Both articles suggest that women and midwives need to be freer, rather than more constrained, about how and with whom they birth. We need to consider the possibility of more rather than fewer ways of training and practising in order to meet the increasingly diverse needs of women and midwives. In order for this to happen, we need to craft a future in which maternity services are valued enough to be properly structured and resourced, to enable birth and midwifery to flourish again.

References

AIMS (2011) 'International witch hunt: the campaign against midwifery'. *AIMS Journal* 23 (3).

Beech, B. (1985) 'Imagine a caesarean section'. *AIMS Quarterly Journal* Late Summer: 14.

Davies, L., Daellenbach, R. and Kensington, M. (eds) (2011) *Sustainability, Midwifery and Birth*. London and New York: Routledge.

Davis-Floyd, R., Faber, M. and De Vries, R. (2013) 'An update on the Netherlands'. *Midwifery Today*: 105: 55–59.

Donnison, J. (1988) *Midwives and Medical Men: A History of the Struggle for the Control of Chilbirth*. New Barnet and London: Historical Publications.

Edwards, N.P. (2005) *Birthing Autonomy: Women's Experiences of Planning Home Births*. London: Routledge.

Hogg, C. and Williamson, C. (2001) 'Whose interests do lay people represent? Towards an understanding of the role of lay people as members of committees'. *Health Expectations* 4: 2–9.

Kirkham, M. (2013) 'Modern birth: processes and fears'. *Midwifery Matters* 136: 3–6.

Leboyer, F. (1975) *Birth without Violence*. London: Fontana.

M4M (2013) 'A midwife for me and my baby'. http://www.m4m.org.uk/. Accessed August 2013.

Nolan, M. (2011) *Home Birth: The politics of difficult choice*. New York and Oxon: Routledge.

Reed, B. and Walton, C. (2009) 'The Albany midwifery practice', in R. Davis-Floyd, L. Barclay, J. Tritten and B.A. Daviss (eds), *Birth Models that Work*. London: University of California Press, pp. 141–58.

Squire, J. (1984) 'Selfish mothers?' *AIMS Quarterly Journal* Autumn: 3.

Stewart, N. (1983) 'Confessions of a thwarted midwife'. *AIMS Quarterly Journal* Autumn: 4&8.

Stewart, N. (1989) 'A great gulf'. *AIMS Quarterly Journal.* 1(2): 3.

Stewart, N. (1991) 'What are we AIMing for?' *AIMS Quarterly Journal* 3(1) 1&20.

Stockton, A. (2012) 'The midwife–doula relationship'. *Essentially MIDIRS* 3(1): 32–35.

Williamson, C. (1992) *Whose Standards? Consumer and Professional Standards in Health Care.* Buckingham and Philadelphia: Open University Press.

Walcott, L. (2009) 'Wasn't I just made for this life (I could not *not* be a midwife)?' *Midwifery Matters* 123: 10–12. Also available http://www.midwifery.org.uk/?page_id=535, last accessed 28 July 2013.

Commentary

Nadine's experience of not becoming a midwife expresses a certain amount of frustration but also shows the freedom she has and can continue to enjoy. I was particularly struck by her closing challenges. 'We need to consider the possibility of more rather than fewer ways of training and practising in order to meet the increasingly diverse needs of women and midwives. In order for this to happen, we need to craft a future in which maternity services are valued enough to be properly structured and resourced, to enable birth and midwifery to flourish again'. Here she clearly states that 'one size does not fit all' yet we are increasingly being shoehorned into the sizes that do not fit. With new European Union directives on health professionals being established (as also alluded to by Allison in chapter 4) entry into midwifery programmes is becoming more streamlined. This will possibly lead to the last of the flexibility, that of prior learning, being eroded and women (or indeed men) with life experiences having to return to school and study for elementary qualifications before entering university to undertake their basic midwifery education. Three types of education, an academic programme, an apprenticeship model and a practical training with theoretical input, offered in Canada were reported by Benoit and Davis-Floyd (2004). The researchers concluded that of most benefit to women and to midwives was the practical training. This has not influenced policy makers either in Canada or in other parts of the world, and as more countries move towards academic education without carrying out preliminary research, questions must eventually be raised.

Reference

Benoit, C. and Davis-Floyd, R. (2004) 'Becoming a midwife in Canada: Models of midwifery education', in I .Bourgeault, C. Benoit and R. Davis-Floyd (eds), *Reconceiving Midwifery*. Montreal-Kingston: McGill-Queen's University Press, pp. 169–86.

15

THE EX-MIDWIFE

Elaine Haycock-Stuart

Introduction

I was asked for the first edition to reflect on why I entered midwifery and my recollections of how I experienced midwifery in the late twentieth century, before leaving to become a health visitor. In this second edition chapter, following on from this reflection I utilise a vignette to illustrate why I became an ex-midwife.

How it all began

Why did I decide to become a midwife and then an ex-midwife or rather a health visitor? I decided at a young age (about 7 years) that nursing was the job I wanted to do and I owe much of my continuing desire to nurse to my parents who supported this interest and enthusiasm. There is no family history of the caring professions, yet they valued my choices and respected the work nurses and midwives do. As a child, I was given opportunities to attend the Red Cross and develop first aid skills alongside other such useful things such as lifesaving skills with swimming. At 16 I undertook work experience with school, I was encouraged to look at alternatives to nursing and spent 2 weeks working in a pathology laboratory in the local district hospital. It was enough time for me to be sure that laboratory work was not for me. I recognised that I enjoyed the interpersonal aspects of life, despite being shy, and that a more communicative, humanising experience was important to me. At sixth form college, it was generally accepted that I had decided to nurse and that was that, and there was no careers advice! I was eager to nurse and my family supported the decision.

Nursing

I undertook my nursing education in a large city hospital in the North of England about 90 minutes away from my home. Initially I took time to adapt to being away from home. I made some great friends (several of whom I am still in touch with). I found nursing academically stimulating, yet it was emotionally draining on many occasions. I found myself aged 18 nursing a young woman who was also 18 years old, in a coma following a road traffic accident. Her A level results came through and she had three straight As! Such sadness and heartbreak for the family. I felt this side of nursing work was emotionally challenging, but being able to care for such ill people and supporting their families was a valuable role and most of the time a rewarding role.

As a nurse I found myself being attacked by men in the hospital wards in a state of confusion post myocardial infarction; one hurled a fire extinguisher at me! It was the humour of the other patients and my co-students that got me through much of the turmoil. There was not always a funny side to everything, but when there was, it was important to see it. I was a good hospital nurse – so I am told, I even won a prize or two, but in my nursing programme I enjoyed my community midwifery and health visiting experience and felt this was where I would like to focus my career.

I made the decision that the 'real world' was where I wanted to work, not in the hospital environment. I enjoyed meeting and speaking with people on their terms – usually in their own homes or occasionally at the general practice surgery. I made plans for further education to become a health visitor, but several people I spoke with then back in the 1980s, health visitors and nurses, advised me to gain experience as a midwife before considering health visiting. I respected this advice as it came from several experienced people and I applied for midwifery education. I was successful in obtaining a place in the same hospital where I had become a nurse.

Becoming a midwife

The nursing and midwifery programmes were worlds apart. I had enjoyed my nursing course, but loved my midwifery course! I was not just stimulated, I was challenged. The integration of theory and practice, the clinical rotations; it was very alive and happening. I really had to stay on top of the academic work which was assessed every couple of weeks by class exam. I had to integrate my theory knowledge daily with my clinical practice and be prepared to move every few weeks to a different clinical area of midwifery – labour ward, antenatal ward, postnatal ward, community and neonatal high dependency. It was a fantastic time.

The things I value

Midwifery's strength, in my view, lies in its focused nature on the mother and newborn baby – the specificity of the midwifery work with women during pregnancy, during birth and immediately after, enables midwives to become knowledgeable and skilled in great depth. I considered myself and other midwives to have relatively narrow but deep knowledge and skills as the work is so focused, as opposed to broad and superficial knowledge and skills which I associate with nursing. As a midwife, I felt I knew a great deal about caring for maternal health during pregnancy, labour and postnatally, in addition to foetal development and care of the newborn baby up to 28 days. This clarity of role and function was, and still is to me, one of the best things about midwifery.

Reflecting on midwifery, I am usually drawn to the sensational, rarer, significant events, as these seem to make up most of my memories from my midwifery career. The more regular and everyday experiences are less remarkable, but not in any way mundane. However, these daily experiences are not my main reflections on midwifery; it is often the more remarkable events that I dwell on. For this reason, I will reflect on midwifery the way I see it, through the sensational, more than the routine. This is not necessarily how other working midwives would describe or reflect on their current work.

Sensational times

Below I give some reflections on being involved in midwifery care; I have mentioned how difficult it is to reflect in an unbiased way on midwifery work and how easy it is to be drawn to the sensational. It is also important to appreciate that as an ex-midwife I am reflecting on a dynamic profession and my reflections are on a service in the late twentieth century. I know there are similarities with the current context, but there are also vast differences and what I am reflecting on is not necessarily how it is today.

VIGNETTE

Imagine: The Labour Ward

New Year's Eve, night shift and the delivery suite (labour ward) is frantically busy with women in labour and family members providing support. I am supporting a couple expecting their first baby, the wife is there in the throes of the birth. I am prepared for the arrival of a new baby when the father faints and bangs his head on the floor – the accident book will have to wait! The mother is the one who needs supporting with this birth! The father will have to wait. Happily a 'normal' birth, no complications – except I have to complete the accident book for the father who fainted and fell and now has a big bump on his head.

Half an hour later and minutes from midnight and I am supporting another couple expecting their first baby – the father has declared he has no desire to be present at the actual birth. I cannot find another member of staff who is not completely involved in a birth elsewhere – no midwife, no auxiliary, and no student! I need a hand, this is a big baby, the mother is tall, but when all is said and done, this is a BIG baby. I ask the dad just to give a hand as much as he can? Gently, he is coaxed by the mother and me to help support her through the birth, helping her with her breathing, supporting and massaging her back. Thankfully he is looking less stressed and more like he might start to enjoy being at the birth – I reassure him that I am hopeful I will have help from a colleague at the actual birth. The progress is fast and the baby is ready to be born; it is just after midnight! We might get the first New Year Day baby!! (Every year we have a 'little competition' between the other city hospital and ourselves as to which will have the first baby of the year). Not going too smoothly – this baby is big, the head has crowned, but there is shoulder dystocia (the upper body is more difficult to deliver) and the clock is ticking. Sister pops her head round 'can I give a hand?' she asks. Our eyes meet and she comes straight in to help. 'Come on baby, come on baby, come!' Thankfully this 10-pound baby has a safe, normal birth. Even dad is looking happy. It turns out we didn't get the first baby of the year though! Time for a cup of tea I think.

It is not so long before a mother who is in labour with her third child (she has two children which she delivered normally) arrives with her husband. Third baby; this indicates she could be progressing fast and be ready to deliver. I examine the mother and listen to the foetal heart – the baby's heart rate is slow – much too slow at 45 beats per minute! (A normal heart rate is about 120–160 beats per minute and a low heart rate suggests a lack of oxygen for the baby). I ask the mother to turn on to her side and explain that she and the baby would benefit from a little oxygen. They are a very calm couple and I am grateful for that. The oxygen has made no difference – the heart rate is very slow. I excuse myself from the couple for a few minutes and go directly to sister; calmly I explain quietly about what I have assessed and the actions I have taken. 'Are you certain it is the foetal heart and not the maternal pulse you are listening to? Have you given her oxygen?' she asks as we both walk back to the couple. We both know this is serious and my recording the maternal pulse in error of the baby's would be something of a relief as it would indicate the baby is in better shape than I think it is, but I know I have made no error and that this mother's pulse is actually faster than her baby's – this woman needs to be in theatre right now and they are full. I had hoped a third baby would be a lovely, straightforward, normal birth without too long to wait. This is not going to happen. Sister examines the woman and listens to the baby's heart rate. She speaks reassuringly to the couple, but explains this baby needs to be delivered in theatre. Sister stays with the couple as I head to prepare for theatre – we usually act as scrub nurse for our own operative deliveries. I speak with the senior registrar in theatre and let him know we have a very urgent need for him to be ready to move straight onto another caesarean section. I explain the circumstances to him and he acknowledges the gravity and urgency of the mother waiting. He is rapidly outside assessing the mother and within minutes she is in theatre; the husband has to wait patiently outside theatre as this is an emergency caesarean – not planned and we sense there is a complication. The baby is delivered gently, the cord is wrapped around the neck twice! The baby would not have survived a normal birth. Mother and baby are both well.

Here I am reflecting on the sensational, but this is very much the reality of life in the labour ward. Yes, there is a great deal of monitoring and waiting, but it is an exciting and stressful place to work too. No two days were the same, but I did have some days when I did not attend a baby's birth and spent a great deal of time monitoring and supporting women only for them to give birth on the next shift. This could be disappointing, but I enjoyed supporting women in labour too and other days could see me attending two or three babies' births.

What is it all about?

Here I offer some reflections on my observations of acute setting midwifery within different contexts and environments. These reflect the kinds of things that I was involved with in midwifery, although I do not feel I had many 'typical' days as most were quite special.

Labour ward

The work in the labour ward could be diverse; for example, supporting or running in theatre for a woman having a caesarean section, attending a woman having a normal birth or monitoring a woman in early labour, as just a few examples. Occasionally a woman may need support giving birth to a stillborn baby or a doctor may need the midwife to assist with a forceps or complicated delivery and support the woman. There is a great variety in how women labour and the nature of support they and their families need during labour.

They say variety is the spice of life and I feel this is particularly true for me when I worked in the labour ward or delivery suite. For me every birth was different – the dynamics of very different women and partners make it so. Then you have the different ways people 'progress' during labour and how they eventually give birth to the baby and the responses they have to a new baby as well as the different health outcomes of each newborn baby. Many factors influence this very dynamic process in the labour ward and there is really very little that I, on reflection, would call 'typical' about it.

Antenatal ward

Some women may be in the antenatal ward to rest, be monitored, have further investigations for the management of a complicated pregnancy such as a low-lying placenta, for example, or in advance of a planned caesarean section for a breech baby; others may be hospitalised as a result of an illness such as unstable diabetes or require specific nursing care in relation to a medical condition. As a midwife I would be caring for women with very different needs and some women would spend a considerable length of time hospitalised, within the ward, whereas others might only be there a day or two. Some women would require high levels of nursing and personal care and others might be closely monitored but independent.

Many women in antenatal wards are concerned about other dependents and family members at home and rarely are women in the antenatal ward happy to be there! Some women were unhappy about their hospitalisation and often felt well in themselves and they really wanted to be home, but were hospitalised for lengthy periods. I often had the feeling that the antenatal ward had parallels with a prison for some women and that they hoped for the great escape. Often as a midwife I felt I was viewed more as a jailer by some women – encouraging them to rest – than a supportive midwife. The women wanted to be home with their families and my observation of them and their foetus were all that stood in their way from escaping!

An interesting observation about midwives and antenatal wards is that although midwives normally only conduct normal births, every woman on an antenatal ward anticipates a potentially complicated delivery. I always find this something of a paradox. Midwives need to know such a great deal about 'abnormal' pregnancy, but usually only conduct deliveries which are normal – admittedly they give support to complicated births too! As a midwife on an antenatal ward I felt that most of the women I was caring for were unlikely to have a normal birth, yet we undertook a great deal of antenatal care with them. When these women did come to give birth it was often another labour ward midwife who would be present to support the woman and the doctor, not usually the midwife who had cared for her during a lengthy antenatal ward stay. This was often disappointing for the mothers and the antenatal ward midwives who had developed a trusting, caring relationship. Arguably, the antenatal midwife would be better able to support mothers they have cared for during a complicated delivery.

Postnatal ward

Work on the postnatal ward involved helping mothers wishing to breast feed and to develop bonding strategies and childcare skills, for example, feeding, bathing, changing and bonding through touch and eye contact and singing. I would help prepare the mothers for caring for themselves and their baby independently on discharge. I would examine the mothers and their babies to ensure everything was normal.

The postnatal ward is usually a happy place, but sometimes people have complicated deliveries or babies become unwell and this requires the midwife to be skilful in their observations and communications with mothers and families. Mothers can also feel quite low after the birth, yet feel they are under family or peer pressure to be happy at the new birth. Some parents struggle to adapt in the early days to caring for a new baby and sometimes babies are 'unwanted' or are to be adopted. The postnatal environment is complex and no assumptions should be made about how women feel and respond to babies after childbirth as this is a very personal experience and requires skills of observation and sensitivity on the part of midwives to support mothers after delivery.

VIGNETTE

Moving on

It is late evening as we come towards the end of a late shift and I am in the nursery on the postnatal ward talking with the two nursery nurses who have worked here for many years (I had moved to Scotland the previous year and secured work as a midwife in a busy city hospital). As we feed and change babies whose mums are resting, one asks me about my decision to leave midwifery. 'Why are you going?' Earlier in the week I informed the ward staff that I will be going to study to become a health visitor in the autumn. It seems it came as a great surprise to staff; the senior house officer had said to me 'You are the last person I would have expected to leave. You are so together here.'

In truth I am a little uncertain about my decision. I came into midwifery with the ultimate aim of becoming a health visitor. I have enjoyed my midwifery education and staffing immensely. I have stayed longer than I needed, but I have really enjoyed it so much I did not envisage leaving to become a health visitor again until I moved to Scotland. Should I let a few frustrations force me out? Are they really just a few frustrations or are they really something really quite big and problematic?

I came to Scotland and took a while to adjust to the climate, but that was not the only reason for me often feeling low in those first few months. At work, when I first arrived I was handed a cardboard box and informed that that was the resuscitation equipment for the babies! I was mortified, this was primitive! On a subsequent occasion I asked about gloves for examining the mothers and babies – none were supplied and when I started ordering them, I was reprimanded for the cost implications. I was working in a city with high rates of HIV, but I seemed to be the only person concerned about the midwives' welfare in respect of the transmission of infection.

I started taking blood when it was required by the doctors (I had been trained to do this down south) and again I was reprimanded – 'midwives do not do that on this ward'! When I did take blood I had to draw it up by syringe and squirt it into containers. I had been used to the syringes which you snapped the needles off and sent the syringe to the laboratory for investigation, to reduce spillage of blood and transmissions of infection. Several things made me feel I had stepped back in time 10 years!! (Life on Mars: the Midwifery Story? Perhaps not!) Eventually I was asked to help teach some of the other midwives and students how to take blood; it was good to see progress.

I had asked several times to be allowed to rotate to a different clinical area during my year here on the postnatal ward, but this has not been granted and I had been advised it would be a considerable length of time before I could expect to move to another area. Occasionally I have been moved briefly to help in a different clinical area if they are short staffed, but I was rarely moved. Are these good reasons for moving on? I think so and I explain to the nursery nurses why, for these kinds of reasons, I am going.

'It is a big shame for us. We will be sad to see you go' they reply. I am surprised by their comment and I ask them why? They explain to me their observations; apparently I am the only staff midwife that allocates myself mothers and babies when I am in charge of the ward, so it evens out the workload amongst more staff. The other staff midwives take no mothers or babies, but stick with managerial work only, for example, the ward round and medicine round. I had never noticed this, but it matters to the nursery nurses; to them it shows I care about the clinical care, not purely wanting to manage. It also shows I share the work more equitably. It seems many of my colleagues are not continuing with the hands-on clinical contact with mothers and babies when they are in administrative charge. I wonder why this would be so. I know being in charge has managerial commitments, but I always combine these with clinical work. Sometimes I ask colleagues to keep a close eye on 'my' mothers and babies for a brief time if I am involved heavily in a managerial aspect of work, but I do not absolve myself from clinical responsibilities and clearly my colleagues value this approach. This just reaffirms to me that I need to move on. I do not want to start adopting the same purely managerial approach to my work. I enjoy working with the mothers, but really do not enjoy the constraints on my professional sphere of practice and future professional development. I have made the right decision – I think.

Looking back

Initially as a qualified midwife, my work was diverse and the 3-monthly rotations in the first city hospital I worked in meant I felt capable of moving into different clinical areas of midwifery with relative ease and little anxiety – we would rotate through the labour ward and antenatal/postnatal ward about every 12 weeks. A typical day is hard to define as each area was so very different. A typical day in the labour ward was not the same as a typical day in an antenatal ward or a postnatal ward. Variety and change was brilliant and I think one of the strengths of midwifery. I had less opportunity to rotate through clinical areas when I moved to Scotland and spent a year in the postnatal ward. I considered this deskilling and was frustrated at the lack of opportunity to rotate through the clinical areas amongst other things, and this was a main driver for me moving out of midwifery and into health visiting. I had primarily entered midwifery in preparation for becoming a midwife and I turned to health visiting when I became dissatisfied with the organisational infrastructure for midwifery in the hospital I worked in.

Was health visiting a good choice?

In truth, midwifery and health visiting are worlds apart and it would take a further chapter – possibly a book – to fully reflect on my experiences of health visiting, but midwifery was valuable within my subsequent work as a health visitor. I am not convinced, though, that midwifery is essential to becoming a health visitor as many people led me to believe. There are aspects of midwifery which without a doubt have helped me in my subsequent work as a health visitor, but there is much more it did not prepare me for. Health visiting too has evolved dramatically in the last 20 years and in reality the work now is different to when I first commenced health visiting; child protection is now a main feature of health visiting work and midwifery does not prepare you well for this. I eventually left health visiting and clinical practice following doctoral studies as there was and still is a lack of opportunity for clinical research careers, despite the rhetoric and the policy development in this area. I am now a Senior Lecturer using my nursing, midwifery and health visiting experience in an academic research career.

Conclusion

I enjoyed midwifery in both the hospital and the community and worked a variety of shifts, for example, evenings and nights as well as morning shifts. There are now assessment units for midwives to further use their skills. Midwifery work is varied, interesting and valuable; it is a dynamic environment where I learned to enjoy 'change' which I think has been of great benefit to me in my subsequent career.

My reflections beg the question – why would you want to leave something you enjoyed so much? There are a few reasons and all are related to the organisation of midwifery in the late twentieth century and are not necessarily the same now. For me midwifery needs regular rotation, not necessarily every 12 weeks, but at least every 6 months. I was unable to be guaranteed a rotation of any kind when I moved to Scotland. Some of the extended roles I undertook in England were not permitted in Scotland at the time and I felt I was being deskilled. Promotion within midwifery looked limited and although I did not realise it at the time, I was ambitious. I began to feel midwifery was shrinking around me as I became limited to the postnatal clinical area, inhibited in the clinical skills I could practise and saw promotion as a very distant point on a very long horizon. I enjoyed the work, but needed the variety that I had enjoyed earlier in my midwifery career.

I always say I would go back to midwifery given half a chance because I remember it fondly, enjoyed it and valued the work I did. Jennifer Worth's book *Call the Midwife* (2012) and successful television series demonstrate to me some of the nostalgia that reflection on a bygone time presents. For my birthday this year my family bought me *The Midwife's Here!* (2012) by Linda Fairley, one of Britain's longest serving midwives. Were they trying to tell me something? I love the clear-cut focus of the remit of the midwife with the vast opportunity for variety within that focus. So what holds me back? Today it is still to some extent the reasons given in this chapter, but in addition there is the more personal impact of how midwifery is organised: where is the good 24/7 childcare that women in the caring professions need to work shifts when they have no family support living near by? As a mother of a young child with a partner who works abroad a lot and no family within 240 miles, I could not return to shift work without flexible 24/7 childcare. Midwifery and indeed nursing are female-dominated professions and there needs to be more consideration of family-friendly policies. In the future many of us will be caring for elderly family members. So if we are not caring for children we will probably be looking after an older person. If the National Health Service addressed these issues then maybe I would be less of an ex and more of a midwife.

References

Fairley, L. (2012) *The Midwife's Here!* London: Harper Element.
Worth, J. (2012) *Call the Midwife*. London: Phoenix.

Commentary

Elaine's journey mirrored many of the time; to become a midwife one had first to become a nurse, and to become a health visitor one had to be both a nurse and midwife, often with a Certificate in District Nursing thrown into the mix. Nowadays things are a bit more streamlined but this poses the question would Elaine ever have become a midwife if she were planning on health visiting today? That question cannot of course be answered, but one thing is certain: had she not had the practice as a midwife that she documents in this chapter, she would have missed out on a substantial part of life's experience. Elaine writes of her doubts and uncertainties about moving on, again something that will resonate with many readers. However, it is clear that she relishes a challenge and has made the most of each new situation.

I wonder, however, if there is such a thing as an 'ex-midwife' and if so just what does it mean? Possibly Elaine is no longer registered with the UK's Nursing and Midwifery Council as a midwife. This means that she should not practise as a midwife in the UK, but does it mean that she no longer has any midwifery skills? Somehow I suspect this is not the case, that those skills which she learned and developed as a midwife, she has brought with her first to health visiting and then to her work as a lecturer. It is impossible to shake off the shackles and once a midwife, always a midwife!

16

CONCLUSION

Valerie Fleming and Rosemary Mander

This book puts together the thoughts of midwives in various practice situations; those who are employed in the communities, in hospitals and in the academic world, as well as those who practise independently and those who embrace more than one of the practice fields. In addition, midwives working in three countries, the United Kingdom, the Netherlands and Switzerland have contributed, so bringing a wider spectrum of ideas to the succeeding pages. Looking further at the individual authors' biographies, it is clear that their professional experience extends well beyond the traditional expectations of becoming a midwife.

This book has sought to provide some answers to the question 'why become a midwife?' For those readers who are thinking of becoming midwives the chapters that form this book may well challenge them even before they start as they think 'all I want to do is to help women give birth'. Conversely, experienced midwives seeking a change may think 'well, why have they chosen these options? There could be more.'

To the first group of people, we hope we have given a small flavour of what this profession has to offer. In Chapter 6, Jean writes about the BBC series *Call The Midwife* provoking an increase in applications from people interested in becoming midwives. However, *Call The Midwife* was set in the 1950s in one area of the UK and practice no longer resembles what is portrayed there. Or does it? As indicated in various chapters of this book the midwife needs to be capable of multi-tasking, using all her senses, developing relationships and providing safe and competent care. It seems that the midwives portrayed in the popular series use exactly the same skills. It is, thus, the settings that have changed rather than the art of midwifery. This necessitates a different education and a deeper awareness of research findings that underpin the latest developments in practice. In Chapters 7 and 13 the need for carrying out and publishing research has been stressed but it is also vital that the midwife is able to evaluate research from other professional groups with a critical eye so that she can accept or reject the findings in her own practice with confidence. One example of non-research-based practice is that of active management of labour, which was widely introduced in developed countries in the 1970s. Its effects are still being felt. but when its various components are unpicked and traced back to their origins, many do not come from a sound research base but possibly only drew on an economic model reducing childbearing to a conveyor belt mentality. Every chapter of this book shows the human element and reflects the joy midwives experience in their daily work.

Those midwives questioning why we chose the topics of the book pose a different challenge. The answer is complex. First we tried to cover the whole spectrum of childbearing because for many onlookers (and we suspect midwives too!) 'real midwifery' only takes place in the labour ward. Sadly, in many countries this is indeed the case as, due to shortage of numbers, midwives are concentrated in this setting so leaving essential ante- and postnatal care in the hands of nurses. In Chapter 4, Allison alludes to the decreasing number of postnatal visits allocated to women once they are discharged from hospital if they are experiencing no complications. However, she also points out that it is only with regular monitoring visits to well women that complications will be detected and treated before they become serious, necessitating further costly stays in hospital. The converse is also true in some parts of the world in which doctors are the mainstay in labour wards where they are assisted by health care assistants or other less well trained personnel. Even more challenging perhaps is the rise in popularity of epidural anaesthesia which in some cases has led to a decline in monitoring of women's labour by midwives. We are well aware of these issues and have sought to provide a rounded view of the midwife's role in a variety of settings as well as spanning the spectrum of childbirth. The example of perinatal mental health in Chapter 5 illustrates one aspect which is a developing speciality role for midwives. Equally, we could have chosen midwives working with younger or older childbearing women, with immigrant women, with those women suffering from perinatal loss or with those women with highly complex medical problems amongst others. To include all would have been impossible.

That leaves us with the question 'Just what is midwifery?' It is generally accepted that in the English language mid-wife derives from the Anglo-Saxon, *mid* meaning with and *wife* meaning 'woman'. If we accept this definition, and most midwives would do so without any difficulty, then the word midwife actually is more appropriate to be a verb rather than a noun as it describes the actions a person would take. However, it is interesting to note that in other languages the word for midwife describes the person herself. In German she is a 'Hebamme', the older woman who lifts the child up from the floor, assuming, very sensibly, that women give birth from a vertical position, and in Danish she is 'Jordmodern' (earth mother). In Slovenian she is a 'babica' (grandmother, a respected elder woman) and in French a 'sage-femme' (wise woman). These have similar connotations to the German but even languages which are unrelated to those of present-day western Europe have similar meanings. The Arabic word for example is 'Qabelah' meaning an able woman who receives the baby. In the Maori language a midwife is a 'Kaiwhakawhānau', literally the controller of the direction of the family. So while the English word seems to be more of an action statement than those of the other languages it makes an interesting contrast.

Perhaps it is through the English word that the well known World Health Organization's (2005) International Definition of the Midwife came about in which the 'midwife is a person who, having been regularly admitted to a midwifery educational programme, duly recognised in the country in which it is located, has successfully completed the prescribed course of studies in midwifery and has acquired the requisite qualifications to be registered and/or legally licensed to practise midwifery.' That implies that the midwife is well educated, a point which has been stressed directly in Chapters 1 and 7 and indirectly in all of the others. In the UK and many other countries, that education now takes place in the academic setting, with a university degree now being the minimum standard for entry to practice. However, a degree on its own cannot guarantee safe practice and in Chapter 6 the safeguards employed in the UK are spelt out. A country which has taken this further than the UK is New Zealand, which has set up a model of peer review based on an inherent partnership of the woman and the midwife. This model ensures an annual review of all midwives' practice with a deeper review taking place triennially and certificates of competence to practise only being awarded on completion of a successful review process.

In essence, then, this book focuses on what being a midwife in certain settings really is about. The vignettes paint vivid pictures of the realities of the individual authors, some of whom have been practising midwives for many years while others, such as Kirsty, are at the beginning of their professional life and have a lot to offer in midwifery's future development.

Midwifery has much to be proud of but equally has much to do if the visibility won in recent years through media exposure is to be maintained. The constantly increasing rate of caesarean sections in the industrialised countries, for example, is a hotly debated topic in both public and professional fora. Some see birth by caesarean section as a safe, predictable and effective preventive alternative to unpredictable vaginal birth, while others claim it as economically driven, with unacceptably adverse effects on the health of both mother and infant. The World Health Organization's recommended rate of 10–15 per cent to ensure optimal care (Moore 1985) includes caesarean sections carried out on purely medical grounds when vaginal birth is not possible and the surgical procedure is required to prevent harm to the woman and/or infant. In cases such as maternal fear of giving birth, other forms of intervention may be possible to achieve the best outcomes. This advice remains unchanged two decades later (Gibbons et al. 2010). Yet high-quality midwifery research in this area is lacking and indeed midwives' voices are often lacking from the professional debates. Midwives need to stand up and be counted in situations like this or our future could be limited as we are replaced by technology.

However, let us end on a positive note and to do this it seems appropriate to return to New Zealand where midwifery almost became extinct 30 years ago. It was the combined efforts of women and midwives that turned it into the dynamic, thriving profession that it is today. Hopefully, readers of this book will feel similarly energised to challenge present practices that are incompatible with their own views of midwifery and ensure a better future for both women and the profession of midwifery.

References

Gibbons, L., Belizán, J., Lauer, J., Betrán, A., Merialdi, M. and Fernando, A. (2010) 'The global numbers and costs of additionally needed and unnecessary caesarean sections performed per year: overuse as a barrier to universal coverage'. Geneva: World Health Report (2010) Background Paper, 30.
Moore, B. (1985) 'Appropriate technology for birth'. *Lancet* 326 (8458), 787.
WHO (2005) *International Definition of the Midwife*. Geneva: World Health Organization.

GLOSSARY

Amni-hook
A disposable instrument used to rupture the membranes (See ARM below. Smyth *et al.* 2007).

ARM
Artificial rupture of membranes (or amniotomy), an intervention by midwives and others intended to augment or accelerate labour (Smyth *et al.* 2013).

CTG
Cardiotocograph, an electronic device to monitor uterine contractions and the fetal response to them.

Elective
A phenomenon which is chosen, but often used to mean a caesarean which is planned, as opposed to an emergency operation. In this context the term gives no indication of who makes the plans or the reason for the caesarean.

Flat
A newborn baby suffering from respiratory depression.

HDU
High Dependency Unit, the area where care is provided for women with serious health problems.

Keys
Usually refers to the keys (among others) of the controlled drugs cupboard. These keys are ordinarily carried by the midwife in administrative charge of the ward or unit, so they may carry some symbolic significance. The midwife 'in charge', though, will give the keys to any midwife needing to administer a controlled drug.

Multigravida

A woman having her second or subsequent baby.

ME

Myalgic encephalomyelitis – commonly known as CFS or Chronic Fatigue Syndrome.

OP

Occipito posterior position, a position of the fetal head in the mother's pelvis which is associated with a long labour.

Paed

Paediatrician.

PPH

Post partum haemorrhage, serious bleeding, usually via the vagina, after the birth of the baby.

Synto

Syntocinon, a synthetic form of the naturally occurring posterior pituitary hormone oxytocin, which (among other effects) causes uterine contractions.

OR (depending on the context)

Syntometrine, a combination of Syntocinon (see above) and ergometrine, a similar oxytocic substance. Syntometrine is widely used in the active management of the third stage of labour (McDonald *et al.* 2004).

References

McDonald, S.J., Abbott, J.M. and Higgins, S.P. (2004) 'Prophylactic ergometrine-oxytocin versus oxytocin for the third stage of labour'. *Cochrane Database of Systematic Reviews*, Issue 1. Art. No.: CD000201. doi: 10.1002/14651858.CD000201.pub2.

Smyth, R.M.D., Alldred, S.K. and Markham, C. (2007) 'Amniotomy for shortening spontaneous labour'. *Cochrane Database of Systematic Reviews*, Issue 4. Art. No.: CD006167. doi: 10.1002/14651858.CD006167.pub2.

Smyth, R.M.D., Markham, C. and Dowswell, T. (2013) 'Amniotomy for shortening spontaneous labour'. *Cochrane Database of Systematic Reviews*, Issue 6. Art. No.: CD006167. doi: 10.1002/14651858.CD006167.pub4.

INDEX